J. Gerard Loeber and Carla G. van El

Forty Years of Heel Prick Screening in the Netherlands

The publication of this book is sponsored by

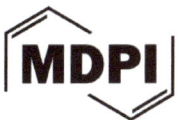

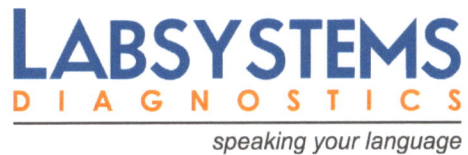

MDPI

LABSYSTEMS
DIAGNOSTICS
speaking your language

Authors
J. Gerard Loeber
Bilthoven
Netherlands

Carla G. van El
Free University Medical Centre in Amsterdam
Netherlands

Editorial Office
MDPI AG
Klybeckstrasse 64
Basel, Switzerland

Publisher
Shu-Kun Lin

1. Edition 2016

MDPI • Basel • Beijing • Wuhan • Barcelona

ISBN 978-3-03842-189-4 (Hbk)
ISBN 978-3-03842-190-0 (PDF)
ISBN 978-3-03842-191-7 (EPUB)

Original Edition: ISBN 978-90-8562-133-1
Prelum Publishers, Houten, The Netherlands

Preface

Sometimes a healthy baby is born, but in the first months or years of life a serious problem may become apparent, such as developmental delays. Parents who were over the moon right after delivery, start getting worried. They often search a long time for a diagnosis. Sometimes such a developmental delay can be prevented by timely use of a diet or a drug. By investigating all new born babies, a diagnosis can be made even before the first symptoms become noticeable.

In the past fifty years, there have been rapid technological advances that facilitated the diagnosis and treatment of a number of metabolic diseases and endocrine disorders. These developments raised and continue to raise many questions, from "Should mothers of healthy newborns approve that their baby's blood is taken?" to "Do we want everything that is technically possible?" or "What are the limits of preventive health care?". The paediatricians, Health Council and parent and patient organisations formed their opinion and advised the minister. A nationwide screening programme was developed to quickly analyse a little blood in a lot of children. An extensive programme of informing (future) parents, visits mostly at home with parents and newborns by primary care nurses, laboratories with high throughput equipment, reporting of adverse results through local paediatricians or family doctors and follow-up in hospitals by (often specialized) paediatricians. A dynamic teamwork with many stakeholders. Over the years, the programme was enhanced by innovations in Information and Communications Technology (ICT), adding new tests, improved information leaflets with professional material, and lessons from abroad.

This book records the history of 40 years of heel prick screening in the Netherlands, from the perspective of Dr. J. Gerard Loeber who for many years was the head of the laboratory of the RIVM (National Institute for Public Health and Environment) that performed the "baby screening" and functioned as a reference laboratory. Gerard Loeber retired in 2012 and in 2013 interviewed many colleagues with whom he had worked for decades. He worked together with Dr. Carla G. van El of the Community Genetics Section (CSG) of the Free University Medical Centre in Amsterdam. She is a sociologist and described the history of genetic screening in the Netherlands in a previous publication.

The start of the story was actually more than 40 years ago, when the first test was invented for the diagnosis of a rare metabolic disease, phenylketonuria (PKU), in blood on filter paper, so that patients could adopt a diet before they developed symptoms. The opportunity to prevent mental retardation was a unique development in public health! Probably it is partly due to the wave of enthusiasm that this created, that led to the implementation of such large organisations in many countries, although initially only a few children did benefit from this. In the Netherlands in the early years it only assisted up to ten children per year, but over the years the number of children diagnosed via the heel prick screening has risen to hundreds each year.

The administrative procedure to invite all children was initially undertaken through the provincial nursing services. The vaccination registries were assigned a role in the heel prick screening. After all, babies were vaccinated in a nationwide programme. Perhaps that explains why sometimes in recent years vaccination is confused with the heel prick. Besides private health care associations, also state institutions were given a new role in the babies care shortly after birth.

This historic book comes at a historic moment. Forty years after the start, a well-functioning Dutch heel prick programme has been developed with the help of the many people involved, providing so many children with a better quality of life. It is time to reflect on what has been built through the efforts of pioneers and all those who contributed their part. At the same time, the programme is facing new challenges: new treatments have become available, and new testing capabilities.

This is a book to help us look back and be proud of what has been achieved, and at the same time to realize that together we can achieve even more for the babies that are born in the Netherlands in the future.

Prof. Martina Cornel
Chair Programme Committee Neonatal Heel Prick Screening
Professor of Community Genetics & Public Health Genomics at the Free Medical Centre in
Amsterdam, Autumn 2014

Structure of the Book

This book aims to provide an overview of developments in the heel prick screening programme in the Netherlands in which similarities with the situation elsewhere in the world, where relevant, will be mentioned. In the Netherlands, the preparations for the national screening programme started in 1964. The formal launch of the programme was on September 1, 1974. In 2014, therefore this programme had existed 40 years.

The book is structured as follows. Chapter 1 describes how the programme began with one disease and over the years has continued to expand to currently covering 19 disorders. Chapter 2 focuses on the organisation of the screening programme and the agencies that have been involved over the years. Chapter 3 is intended to provide a global view of the programme in its current form. Chapter 4 describes how neonatal screening programmes elsewhere in the world developed and outline their main differences with the Dutch programme. Finally, Chapter 5 contains the summary and conclusions. This chosen structure leads to some aspects being mentioned more than once.

The book is intended for a broad audience that is interested in policy making on heel prick screening; hence, scientific depth is limited. Where possible and useful, references to the scientific literature have been included but completeness has not been pursued. The main sources were the archives of the National Steering Committees for Phenylketonuria and Congenital Hypothyroidism (LBCs), supplemented with interviews with the persons listed in Annex 1 and, if available, their personal archives.

The Authors
Autumn 2014

This is a translation of the book "Veertig Jaar Hielprikscreening in Nederland", that was published by Prelum Publishers, Houten, the Netherlands with ISBN 978-90-8562-133-1
© 2014 Prelum, Houten; RIVM, Bilthoven; Vumc, Amsterdam.

The assistance of Mrs Kate Hall, Birmingham, UK, with the translation is greatly appreciated.

The Authors
Autumn 2015

Acknowledgements

During the writing of this book Gerard Loeber was associated as a researcher with the Section of Community Genetics, EMGO+ and Department of Clinical Genetics at the Free University Medical Centre in Amsterdam from 1 January 2013 to 31 December 2013. Carla van El is a researcher in the same section.

This book is the result of the research project "Neonatal screening in the Netherlands: a historical and policy perspective" of the CSG Centre for Society and the Life Sciences, funded by the Netherlands Genomics Initiative. Additional funding was obtained from the Centre for Population Screening, RIVM, Bilthoven. A supervisory committee was formed for this research project.

The text of this book is partly based on interviews with founders of heel prick screening in the Netherlands and current experts in different fields of screening. The authors thank the members of the supervisory committee and all those interviewed very much for their comments and suggestions.

About the Authors

Gerard Loeber studied biochemistry at the University of Amsterdam and received a PhD from the Faculty of Mathematics and Physics at the University of Nijmegen with a thesis on human luteinising hormone. From 1979 to 2012 he was employed in various positions at the RIVM in Bilthoven. Throughout this period he was closely involved with the heel prick screening programme; since 1990 as head of the reference laboratory.

Carla van El studied sociology at the University of Amsterdam and received a PhD from the Faculty of Philosophy at the University of Groningen for a thesis on schools and styles in sociology. With some interruptions she has been employed since 2003 as a researcher at the Section Community Genetics, EMGO+ and Department of Clinical Genetics at the Free University Medical Centre in Amsterdam. Her research focuses on the history and policies of genetic screening.

Table of Contents

List of Abbreviations

The Dutch acronyms have been kept unchanged for clarity and reference; the translation serves only to clarify but may not always be an officially recognised equivalent.

AMC	Academic Medical Centre Amsterdam
ANP	Dutch Press Agency
ANHS	Advisory Committee Neonatal Heelprick Screening
AWBZ	Exceptional Medical Expenses Act
CAH	Congenital adrenal hyperplasia
CF	Cystic fibrosis
CH	Congenital hypothyroidism
CN	Caribbean part of the Netherlands
CPPS	Coordinating Committee Pre- and Post-natal Research Ziekenfondsraad
CvB	Centre for Population Screening—RIVM
CVZ	Health Care Insurance Board
DNA	Deoxyribonucleic acid
DVP	Unit Vaccination and Prevention Programmes—RIVM
GBA	Common Population Administration
GHI	Health Care Inspectorate
JGZ	Youth health care
KNOV	Royal Netherlands Organisation of Midwifes
LAC	National Advisory Committee
LBC	National Steering Committee
LBNS	National Steering Committee Neonatal Screening—CVZ
LHV	National Society of General Practitioners
LUMC	Leiden University Medical Centre
LVE	National Society of Vaccination Registries
LVT	National Society of Home Care
MCADD	Medium-chain acyl CoA dehydrogenase deficiency
MZ	Metabolic diseases
NEORAH	Neonatal Registration Abnormal Heel Prick Screening Results
NIPG	Netherlands Institute for Preventive Medicine
NIVEL	Netherlands Institute for First Line Health Care
NSCK	Netherlands Signalling Centre Paediatrics
NVK	Netherlands Society for Paediatrics
PKU	phenylketonuria
PNHS	Programme Committee Neonatal Heel Prick Screening
RCP	Unit Regional Coordination Programmes—RIVM
RIV	National Institute for Public Health (until 1984)
RIVM	National Institute for Public Health and the Environment (since 1984)
SCID	Severe combined immunodeficiency syndrome
SZ	Sickle cell disease
T4	Thyroxine (=thyroid hormone)

TBG	Thyroxine-binding globulin
Thal	Thalassemia
TNO	Organisation for Applied Scientific Research
TSH	Thyrotropin (=thyroid stimulating hormone)
Radboudumc	Radboud University Medical Centre Nijmegen
UMCG	University Medical Centre Groningen
UMCU	University Medical Centre Utrecht
VUmc	Free University Medical Centre Amsterdam
ZonMw	Netherlands Organisation for Health Research and Development

Introduction

Infants are examined shortly after birth by taking a few drops of blood from the heel. The test results of this blood test, called heel prick screening, may suggest that the child needs a special diet or pharmaceutical drugs to prevent a developmental delay.

In the Netherlands *heel prick screening* is a fairly well known but somewhat artificial term. At first glance, the phrase seems to indicate that the heel prick itself is being screened, as if you look at how that is done, but that is nonsense of course. The heel prick is no more than a technique for the collection of a number of drops of blood from the heel of a newborn baby. Terms like newborn screening or neonatal screening are actually preferable.

Screening is derived from the verb 'to screen', a synonym of the verb 'to sieve', *i.e.*, the sieving out of individuals that you are looking for, from a large group of individuals that you are not interested in. Screening, for example, is used as a term for the process of verifying whether a person is a security risk. If he passes through the sieve, he is OK.

In health care, screening is used for the medical examination of (parts of) the population for certain diseases with the intention to identify persons who might be suffering from one of the diseases. It is an offer supported by the government to an, in principle, asymptomatic population. Through targeted diagnosis the result of the screening is confirmed or denied.

Known examples of screening programmes are those for breast cancer, cervical and colon cancer, but also for congenital anomalies of the foetus during pregnancy, known as prenatal screening.

This book concerns the screening for congenital disorders in newborns, formally designated as 'neonatal screening' but in daily practice as 'heel prick screening in newborns'. The first condition screened for was an inborn metabolic disorder.

Inborn metabolic disorders, originally called 'inborn errors of metabolism', were first described by Archibald Garrod over 100 years ago. They typically involve genetic changes that lead to a reduced or even absent activity of certain enzymes, which in turn are needed for the conversion of components in the blood. If such reactions do not proceed well, there is a build-up of one component and/or a shortage of another component. There are dozens of known metabolic disorders that can result from a variety of causes, of which only some are detected in the heel prick programme. In Garrod's time, one could only conclude that someone suffered from a metabolic disorder but could not treat it, with all the health consequences that entailed.

Garrod himself discovered the mechanism of alkaptonuria, a problem in the conversion of the amino acids, phenylalanine and tyrosine (Garrod 1909). In the following decades it became more and more clear how the metabolic action of enzymes had been disrupted, and what the (patho)physiological effects were. Ivar Asbjørn Følling described the disease phenylketonuria (PKU), a cause of mental retardation, and the occurrence of high concentrations of 3-phenylpyruvate in the urine of such patients, as a result of a build-up of phenylalanine in their blood (Følling 1934).

If it is clear what the defective enzyme is, it seems obvious to administer that enzyme via a diet to fight or prevent the disease. However, enzymes, like other proteins degrade themselves by normal metabolic processes. The alternative is to look at the components that are degraded or produced, respectively, by the enzyme, and to supplement the shortage or to prevent the excess, respectively, by modifying the diet. Horst Bickel in the 1950s reported that a low protein diet, thus with a low phenylalanine intake, had an ameliorative effect on the clinical symptoms of PKU patients.

Also for other metabolic disorders, such as galactosemia, it could be shown that adjusting the diet had an ameliorative effect on the physical condition of the patient.

Much of the above also applies to other groups of diseases that are detected with the heel prick screening, such as diseases with endocrine, haematological or immunological characteristics, where there may be a disorder in the organ's morphology. Thus, for example, a disorder in the thyroid gland is one of the causes of congenital hypothyroidism. In addition to adjusting the diet, medication can sometimes reduce health complaints.

Screening in practice is based on the measurement of the concentration of a marker in the blood (or urine), which is characteristic for the disorder to be screened, and the concentration of which is increased or decreased relative to the normal state. In the ideal case, the concentration of the marker in patients is much higher or lower than in healthy persons. Unfortunately, this is usually not the case and then there is a, sometimes arbitrarily, agreed boundary called the cut-off limit.

Let us take PKU with the marker phenylalanine as an example. If during screening of a child, a very high phenylalanine concentration is found, chances are high that the child is suffering from PKU. If the phenylalanine concentration is only moderately increased relative to the cut-off limit, it could be a mild form of PKU, but also a healthy child that happened to have a high phenylalanine concentration at the time of blood collection. If the cut-off limit is set very high only the real PKU patients are found at screening, but there is a chance that PKU patients who happened to have a slightly lower phenylalanine concentration will be missed. In order not to miss any child, the cut-off limit may be set lower, but that will lead to a number of healthy children with a screen-positive result. During the diagnostic phase it will become clear that these children are healthy and therefore wrongly received a positive screening result, a so-called 'false positive'. In the course of time, more and more data concerning the phenylalanine concentration in real PKU patients as well as in subsequently shown healthy children are collected and the cut-off limit can be determined more accurately.

For some diseases, one marker is insufficient to distinguish between patients and healthy children, and two or more markers are measured. The decision tree is then of course more complicated.

Furthermore, the methodology is sometimes insufficient to solely and exclusively identify the targeted disorders; then also information is obtained about other diseases that are deliberately kept outside the screening programme, or about carriership, a situation in which the child itself is not sick but has a gene variant that is related to a disease. Difficult issues, which in addition to medical aspects, also give rise to complex discussions in view of the ethical and legal aspects.

Chapter 1: The Start and Expansion of the Heel Prick Screening Programme

   Although the Dutch neonatal screening programme was formally started on September 1, 1974, the first discussions and preparations for screening for phenylketonuria started in 1964. The programme was expanded in stages to 19 conditions in 2014. The entire period from 1964 to 2014 can be roughly divided into eight periods:

1. Phenylketonuria (PKU) 1964–1974;
2. Congenital Hypothyroidism (CH) 1975–1981;
3. Consolidation 1981–1995;
4. Congenital Adrenal Hyperplasia (CAH) 1995–2002;
5. MCADD and sickle cell disease 2002–2007;
6. Expansion of panel 2002–2007;
7. Cystic Fibrosis (CF) 2007–2011;
8. Future expansions 2011–2014.

Period 1: Phenylketonuria (PKU) 1964–1974

Developments in the US and England

After Følling's publications in the 1930s (e.g., Følling 1934), in both the US and in England, researchers became interested not only in the disease, but also in methods of detection and treatment.

In the US in 1957, Willard Centerwall published a method for the detection of phenylalanine metabolites in the urine by means of a colour reaction with ferric chloride (Centerwall 1957). This resulted in the first programme being instigated in California as well as in the United Kingdom in which a larger scale of newborn babies were examined with the aid of the urine collected in their diaper. However, this method proved to work well only if the babies were already some weeks old but by then the disease had already caused damage. In addition, some babies showed a positive urine test but still appeared to be healthy. In the 1960s, the first publications by Robert Guthrie (Figure 1.1.) described an alternative method using blood instead of urine (Guthrie 1963).

> *In Phenylketonuria (PKU) the enzyme phenylalanine hydroxylase is absent or in insufficient efficacy. The amino acid phenylalanine that is released during the breakdown of protein in the diet is not properly converted into tyrosine. The high levels of phenylalanine in the blood also leak into the spinal fluid and cause damage to the spinal nerve cells. This ultimately leads to brain damage and mental retardation. PKU patients grow slowly and also have behavioural problems such as aggression and tantrums and many suffer from skin conditions such as eczema that are difficult to treat.*

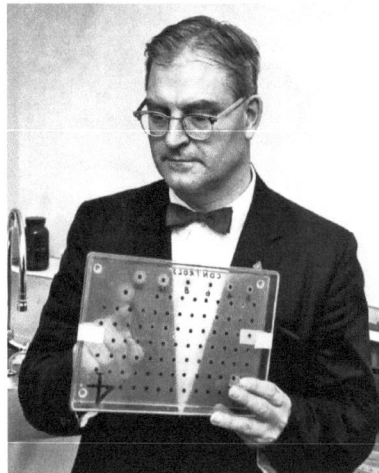

Figure 1.1. Dr. Robert Guthrie shows an agar plate with blood spot punches. The growth zones around certain punches are indicative of an increased phenylalanine concentration.

Dr. Guthrie had earned his fame in scientific cancer research in Buffalo, New York. He had a mentally handicapped son, though not suffering from PKU, but also a niece who was a PKU patient. That was the reason for him joining the Association for Retarded Children (ARC). This group campaigned for the recognition of the existence and the rights of mentally disabled children, which was fairly new in the 1950s. Guthrie noted that the above-mentioned urine test was of insufficient quality. Because of his background in microbiology he experimented with bacterial growth and inhibition, and developed a trusted method that became known as a bacterial inhibition assay or Guthrie test. See Chapter 3 for details.

Introduction of Filter Paper

However, Guthrie's most important achievement was his discovery that the method performed better if the blood had been collected on a piece of filter paper to make it easier to be put on the agar plate (suitable for bacteria to grow) so the blood could not flow out. An important additional benefit was that the filter paper greatly simplified sending blood samples to the laboratory. The final step was then to obtain a blood sample, shortly after birth, via the heel prick.

Guthrie's invention was described in a number of publications in the early 1960s. Initially, he received little recognition, as evidenced by the fact that several scientific journals would not publish his method. Although the patient organisations were enthusiastic, society obviously had to get used to the idea that something could be done about the prevention of mental retardation, while some doctors believed that they themselves were able to detect such handicaps in time. Furthermore, many doctors held little affection for the field of genetics which they regarded to be far removed from their daily practice of diagnosis and treatment. Finally, they considered that a systematic prevention programme implemented by non-medical people was not in concordance with the traditional doctor–patient relationship. However, the Association for Retarded Children (ARC) was aware it had support due to the personal interest of President John F. Kennedy whose sister Rosemary was mentally disabled, and was able to convince the local politicians state by state to make PKU-screening mandatory. Recently, a book has been published about PKU, which deals extensively with this matter (Paul and Brosco 2013).

The first large-scale application took place in the US State of Massachusetts in 1963. That year is also internationally regarded as the beginning of heel prick screening. Starting with screening for PKU only, in the course of the following 50 years, the number of conditions, thanks to increasingly sophisticated techniques, increased to close to 60 in some US states.

Developments in the Netherlands

In the Netherlands, the disease PKU was known (Fleury 1959, Van Sprang 1961), but the children were only clinically diagnosed after mental damage had already occurred. Usually after some time they were placed in homes for the mentally disabled. At that time heel prick screening was as little known in the Netherlands as it was in other countries outside the United States. A paediatric psychiatrist, Dr. J.J.L. ten Brink in Vught had heard about the work of Guthrie at a conference in 1964 in Denmark and had asked Dr. A. Manten, microbiologist at the National Institute of Public Health (RIV) in Bilthoven whether this could be applied in the Netherlands. Dr. Manten sent this letter to the Directorate of the RIV, which ordered Dr. C.E. Voogd, biologist, to verify if the method described by Guthrie could be applied (Manten and Holtz 1964, Manten 1964, Manten and Voogd 1968). Incidentally, according to a letter, dated June 18, 1965, from Dr. J.B.M. Veraart, Chief Health Inspector to the Directorate of the RIV, he had already in 1960 requested attention was paid to these developments in the US; obviously this had been ignored. The Dutch paediatrician, Nelck, published a review article in 1965 about the disease PKU, including the possibilities for screening, diagnosis and treatment (Nelck 1965).

Voogd's research followed two tracks. Firstly, he examined which laboratory method performed better, i.e. the urine test via the already mentioned colour reaction, or the test in blood with the bacterial inhibition assay described by Guthrie. The investigation confirmed the observation in England that the urine test on samples of PKU-patients often show a negative result. It was therefore decided to opt for the bacterial inhibition tests in blood.

> *However, the method still had to be set up. Voogd needed a thousand blood samples from healthy people and ended up at the military medical service. Every year, young men aged 18 had their health check for military service. The colonel on duty did not agree to take a separate blood sample but agreed to Voogd's suggestion to use the blood dripping from the needle to make spots on filter paper. Thus a female RIV laboratorian went along the young men in their underwear, much to the amusement of the people involved.*

Secondly, it was examined how often PKU occurred in the Netherlands in mentally handicapped persons. To this end blood samples from around 22,500 residents in 194 institutions were analysed. In 148 persons, i.e. about 0.7%, the phenylalanine concentration turned out to be increased, which was indicative of the diagnosis of PKU (Manten and Voogd 1968, Anders 1973).

Figure 1.2. shows the first model of a heel prick card. It consisted of a strip of filter paper with places for four blood drops, and was attached to a standard RIV laboratory test request form.

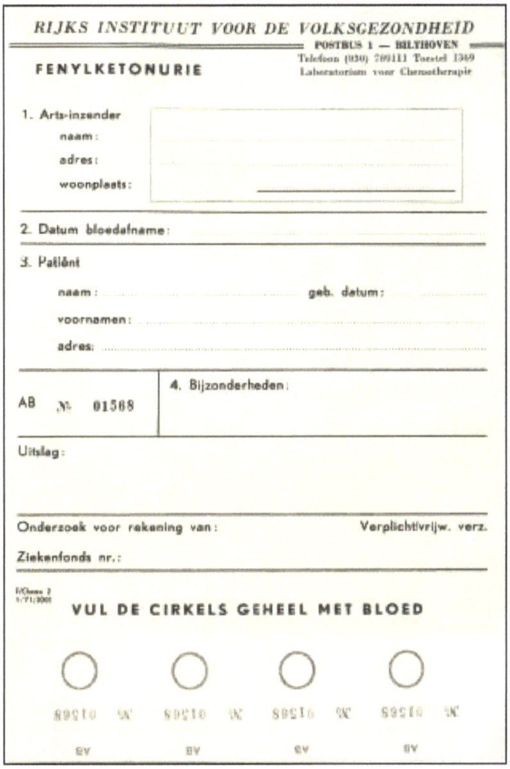

RIJKS INSTITUUT VOOR DE VOLKSGEZONDHEID

POSTBUS 1 — BILTHOVEN
Telefoon (030) 780111 Toestel 1349
FENYLKETONURIE   Laboratorium voor Chemotherapie

1. Arts-inzender
   naam:
   adres:
   woonplaats:

2. Datum bloedafname:

3. Patiënt
   naam: geb. datum:
   voornamen:
   adres:

   4. Bijzonderheden:
AB   N.   01588

Uitslag:

Onderzoek voor rekening van: Verplicht/vrijw. verz.

Ziekenfonds nr.:

VUL DE CIRKELS GEHEEL MET BLOED

○   ○   ○   ○

Figure 1.2. Heel prick card around 1966.

Study Group

The Dutch results, added to reports from other European countries, prompted the then Ministry of Social Affairs and Public Health to set up a study group in 1966. This study group directed a pilot project of neonatal heel prick screening from 1967 onwards. The prevalence (*i.e.* the rate of occurrence) of PKU is higher in the south than in the north of the Netherlands. To gain experience with the detection of PKU patients it would have been more appropriate to carry out the pilot project in the southern provinces of North-Brabant and Limburg. However, this was met with great resistance from the provincial health authorities in those provinces. In contrast, there was interest from the provincial health authorities in the northern provinces, Groningen and Friesland. The choice of these two provinces also had a very practical advantage. The working area of the two northern laboratories from the national network of Regional Laboratories of Public Health, where the analyses were to be carried out, coincided with the provincial borders; this made it simpler in terms of logistics and responsibilities. The registration of the children involved and the screening results were taken care of by the provincial health services (this task was later taken over by the vaccination registries, see Chapter 2). Referral of children with abnormal screening results to a paediatrician was the responsibility of the provincial youth doctors.

The choice of the provincial health services was not undisputed. There were also arguments for involvement of hospitals where all technical aids were available. However, in the 1960s, the percentage of home births was around 60% and these families would then have to go to the hospital with their child shortly after birth, which was expected to lead to a low degree of participation. Unlike in other countries, the Netherlands—probably because of the approach taken—had a participation of more than 99% right from the start. In consultation with the Dutch Paediatric Association it was decided that children with abnormal screening results, in principle, would be referred to academic children's hospitals.

Pilot Screening

The pilot screening started in 1968 under the leadership of Mrs. N. Haverkamp Begemann, provincial paediatrician in Friesland, and would run initially until 1970. Besides a low prevalence of PKU, the selected region also had a relatively small number of births so the probability of detection of PKU patients was small. In 1968, a total of 19,198 children were screened with two abnormal results. One child had had an abnormally high protein intake through the diet which had led to the (false) positive result; the other child had died before diagnostics could confirm the screening results (Study Group Phenylketonuria 1970). The main aim of the pilot screening, however, was the testing of the infrastructure. This process ran so smoothly that it had soon become routine. The project was repeatedly renewed for one year at a time. Therefore, the Court of Audit in 1972 objected because it was felt that with these regular extensions, it could not be regarded as a project anymore and it seemed as if the screening had become a regular service, something which people were entitled to. All this led the Ministry of Health to its decision on a nationwide screening programme. At the urgent request of the Minister, the pilot screening was continued until the national organisation had been implemented. The Health Inspectorate was commissioned to work out procedures and finances (Director General of Public Health 1972). Advice was also sought from the Insurance Council. This body suggested to screen not only for PKU but also for galactosemia. This advice was not adopted because the optimal blood sampling period for PKU (after day 6, day of birth = 0;. Holtzmann *et al.* 1974) would be too late to timely detect galactosemia patients. Incidentally, initially not all senior officials of the Ministry welcomed such a large-scale population research programme. One of the considerations was the hesitance to submit all children and their parents to the trouble (and the pain) of a heel prick to detect a mere handful of affected children. However, in the end, permission was obtained.

Start of Nationwide Programme

In such a screening programme many agencies and professional groups are involved, such as the paediatricians who diagnose PKU cases and treat them, the employees of laboratories, and the people who inform parents and take the blood samples (general practitioners, midwives, staff nursing services, 'screeners'). The study group (then called the Phenylketonuria Working Group) put together a PKU Protocol which was completed in 1973.

In this Protocol, and in the following versions, all daily steps were described including the distribution of responsibilities for those steps in the screening process. In addition, the Inspectorate developed an information brochure about PKU for professionals (GHI, 1974).

Originally it was the decision of the Ministry to start screening by January 1, 1974 (Voogd 1973). This was also the message spread nationally. However, because of budgetary reasons, including amongst others the oil crisis in autumn 1973, it was decided to postpone the start until September 1, 1974. This led to some anxiety at the National Organisation of Mentally Handicapped Care. It advised the parents to have the heel prick carried out by the family doctor, to request the laboratory test themselves and submit the bill to their insurance company (Hermans 1974, National Organisation of Mentally Handicapped Care 1974). It is not clear how many parents did as suggested.

In the text of the decree of the Ministry in June 1974, some details of the implementation were set. The heel prick test had to be performed after at least 5 x 24 hours *post partum* but before the end of the second week of life, and to use laboratory methods to be set by the RIV. The RIV was designated as a 'reference laboratory' and that had never happened before by ministerial decree (Minister V & M 1974). See Figure 1.3.

A reference laboratory has this name because it is considered to have, and to acquire, more knowledge in terms of both content and methodology than the other laboratories involved. The judgments of the reference laboratory in professional disagreements are supposed to be primary. The reference laboratory acts as a sort of *primus inter pares, first among equals*.

MINISTERIE VAN
VOLKSGEZONDHEID
EN MILIEUHYGIENE

Nr. 84614
Afdeling VZ Vgz/Vera

Onderwerp: Besluit uitvoering onderzoek
aangeboren stofwisselingsziekten Bijzondere Ziektekosten
verzekering.

DE STAATSSECRETARIS VAN VOLKSGEZONDHEID EN MILIEUHYGIENE

Gelet op de artikelen 1, vijfde lid, en 3, negende lid, van het Verstrekkingenbesluit
Bijzondere Ziektekostenverzekering 1968 (Stb. 1971, 552)[1];

BESLUIT:

Artikel 1.

Onder onderzoek als bedoeld in artikel 1, eerste lid, onder F van het Verstrekkingenbesluit Bijzondere Ziektekostenverzekering 1968 wordt verstaan een onderzoek naar het
vóórkomen van de stofwisselingsziekte Phenylketonurie (P.K.U).

Artikel 2.

Voor een in artikel 1 genoemd onderzoek komen in aanmerking zuigelingen die de leeftijd
van twee maanden nog niet hebben bereikt en - in zeer bijzondere gevallen - ook oudere
zuigelingen. Een onderzoek dient in de regel plaats te vinden vóór het einde van de
tweede levensweek, doch niet binnen 3 x 24 uur na de geboorte van het betrokken kind.

Artikel 3.

1. Het voor de opsporing vereiste laboratorium-onderzoek wordt uitgevoerd door de
streeklaboratoria voor de volksgezondheid, waarmede het Rijks Instituut voor de
Volksgezondheid te Bilthoven, in dit besluit verder aangeduid als R.I.V., een
contract heeft gesloten.
2. Het in het eerste lid bedoelde laboratorium-onderzoek wordt uitgevoerd volgens de
onderzoekmethoden welke door het R.I.V. worden vastgesteld.
3. Het R.I.V. wordt voor dit laboratoriumonderzoek aangewezen als referentie-instituut.

Artikel 4.

Ingeval een onderzoek als bedoeld in artikel 1 achterwege blijft, neemt het ziekenfonds
de ziektekostenverzekeraar of het uitvoerend orgaan op een door of namens de verzekerd
gedaan verzoek de nodige stappen teneinde te bereiken dat een onderzoek alsnog wordt
verricht.

[1] Laatstelijk gewijzigd bij Koninklijk besluit van 16 mei 1974 (Stb. 323)

- 2 -

Artikel 5.

Dit besluit kan worden aangehaald als Besluit uitvoering onderzoek aangeboren
stofwisselingsziekten Bijzondere Ziektekostenverzekering en wordt in de Neder-
landse Staatscourant geplaatst. Het treedt in werking met ingang van 1 september
1974.

Leidschendam, 26 juni 1974
De Staatssecretaris voornoemd.

w.g. J. P. M. HENDRIKS

Figure 1.3. Decree regarding Inborn Metabolic Diseases.

10

Through publications in various professional journals, the purpose of the screening was explained (Voogd 1974a, b; Bergink 1976; Swaak 1976)). The National Steering Committee PKU, having emerged from the aforementioned working group and headed by Prof. Dr. F.J. van Sprang, paediatrician, reported periodically on the results of the screening (see, for example LBC PKU, 1978, 1981) and also the Inspectorate published a review of the initial results (Verbrugge, 1983). In addition, information material was developed for parents and general practitioners. See Figure 1.4.

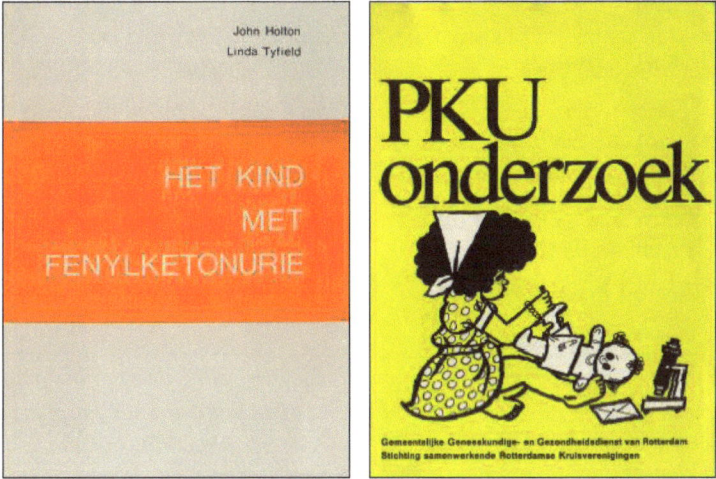

Figure 1.4. Examples of information brochures about PKU.

Period 2: Congenital Hypothyroidism (CH) 1975–1981

International Developments

Congenital hypothyroidism (CH), a thyroid hormone deficiency leading to mental underdevelopment, was first described in detail by Henning Andersen (Denmark) in his thesis in 1960. During a conference in Vienna in 1961 he proposed to get screening started, which was received by the audience with (scoffing) laughter because the idea of a large-scale screening programme for newborns was still unknown. About 10 years later, this idea was picked up in Canada by Jean Dussault and his associates. They had become interested in not only screening the heel prick blood sample for PKU, but also for CH by measuring thyroid hormones. This was made possible by the development of (radio)immunochemical methods (Yalow and Berson 1960), in which very small concentrations, up to millionths of a microgram, of these substances can be measured in the blood (Dussault and Laberge 1973). Early detection of an imbalance of these hormones followed by treatment can prevent CH. CH, like PKU, albeit through a different mechanism, may disrupt the metabolism in brain cells and lead to mental disabilities. PKU can be treated by diet; CH with medications (thyroid hormone).

> *CH is a heterogeneous disease. There may be defects in the thyroid, the pituitary gland or the hypothalamus resulting in an underproduction of the thyroid hormone (T4). If the problem resides in the thyroid the low T4 concentration will stimulate the pituitary gland to make more thyroid stimulating hormone (TSH). This is called primary or thyroidal CH, also known as CH-T, and is therefore characterized by a low T4 concentration and a high TSH concentration. However, if the fault is located in the function of the pituitary gland or the hypothalamus, respectively there is little or no TSH production and also too little T4 produced by the thyroid gland. This is called secondary (resp. tertiary) or central CH, also known as CH-C, and is thus characterized by a (low) normal TSH concentration and a low T4 concentration. CH-C is much less common than CH-T, but detection is of clinical value because usually other pituitary functions are disrupted. In clinical practice, it was revealed that only 11% of children with CH-based features was recognized in time. This screening would therefore be very useful.*

Developments in the Netherlands

The Dutch paediatric endocrinologists, whose main leaders were Prof. Dr. H.K.A. Visser and Prof. Dr. J.L. van de Brande, realised the importance of early detection of CH. In addition to the existing working group PKU, a working group CH was established in 1975 with some of the same staff, but extended with a paediatric endocrinologist and a clinical chemist with expertise in the field of thyroid hormone assays. The working group CH contacted the Inspectorate and the RIV with a proposal for a further pilot project. The Dutch Paediatric Association (NVK) organised a survey among its members to establish interest in such a screening programme. Several laboratories offered to carry out a pilot project. Eventually the

RIV chose the Endocrine Laboratory of the Bergweg Hospital in Rotterdam, led by Dr. W. Schopman, because of his extensive knowledge and experience in the field of endocrinology and the (radio)immunochemistry. Due to the technical and substantive differences with microbiology, the CH-screening could not be simply carried out by the PKU-laboratories.

Pilot Screening

In 1977 the preparations for the trial project, funded by the Praeventiefonds (now ZonMw), started. The pilot project under the inspiring leadership of Prof. Dr. G.A. de Jonge, paediatrician, was carried out in parts of the province of South Holland. The Provincial Health Office of South Holland referred the children detected. The Dutch TNO Institute for Preventive Medicine evaluated not only the results of the screening itself but also of the follow-up diagnostics. To assess what information was relevant, they looked back at the case histories of 95 patients who had been detected clinically in the period 1972–1974. A subsequent project for improvement of diagnostics and follow-up was also approved by the Praeventiefonds.

A formal National Steering Committee CH (LBC-CH) was established by the NVK to oversee the pilot project. The LBC-CH first was headed by Prof. de Jonge, and later by Dr. G. Derksen-Lubsen, paediatrician. The LBC-CH advised the Inspectorate to ask the Ministry to issue a press release to announce the start of the pilot project. Apparently at that time that was not a very obvious action for the Ministry. In the pilot region, much attention was paid to educating the professionals (general practitioners, midwives, paediatricians) and the general public (Derksen-Lubsen and Young, 1978). See Figure 1.5.

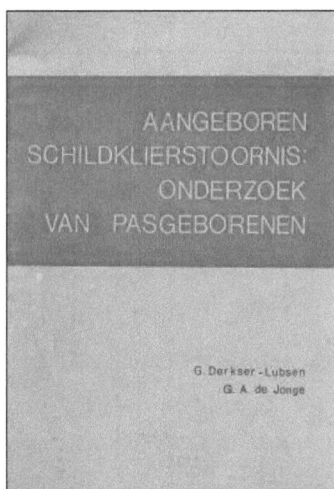

Figure 1.5. Information brochure about thyroid disorders including CH.

In 1978 the actual screening process began in the pilot regions. Through the RIV it became clear that also other clinical chemistry laboratories on their own initiative had started with the determination of thyroid hormone (T4) in blood samples. Although this could have interfered with the pilot the Inspectorate decided not to intervene but to gradually establish the centralisation.

Within the project group, there were heated discussions regarding (a) whether to screen via T4, via TSH, or via a combination of both, one argument being that the determination of T4 was simpler and cheaper; and (b) whether the laboratory analysis was to take place in blood samples that had already been collected for the PKU screening, or in umbilical cord blood. It was more a point of principle. Umbilical cord blood has the advantage that it is available earlier than the heel prick blood samples, but has the disadvantage that the determination of T4 therein is not reliable. Moreover, a separate circuit of blood sampling would have to be introduced, while one also feared that in the rush around childbirth taking a sample of umbilical cord blood could easily be forgotten. Eventually the choice was made for the heel prick blood.

Pressure was exerted on the colleagues involved in the PKU-screening to see whether the heel prick could be performed sooner after birth. At the start of the PKU-screening it had been decided that the heel prick would preferably not be done before the beginning of the second week of life (from day 7, day of birth being counted as 0). At such a time, the child will usually be eating enough so that the protein metabolism reaches a sufficient level. The relatively insensitive Guthrie method would then be able to effectively pick up a disturbance in this metabolism, e.g. in the case of PKU a decreased conversion of phenylalanine into tyrosine, resulting in an increased phenylalanine concentration in the blood. Fortunately around 1990 it became clear from foreign research that classical PKU patients already have an increased phenylalanine concentration after two to three days after birth. However, because the LBC-PKU wished to pick up also the milder forms, it did not want to move the time of the heel prick too much earlier. Eventually, a compromise was agreed to detect both PKU and CH timely and reliably, *i.e.* six to nine days after birth.

During the pilot project, there was frequent contact with foreign colleagues (Dussault, Canada; Delange, Belgium; Illig, Switzerland) who had advanced further in their own countries and who had had similar issues to solve. The recently established European Thyroid Association published the following recommendations.

The optimal timing of blood collection was set to three to seven days after birth, because from that moment the concentrations of the thyroid hormones are relatively stable.

The decision on which of the thyroid hormone (T4 or TSH) to choose as the primary marker for the screening was left to policymakers in each country depending on whether a country wanted to detect only children with thyroidal, primary CH, or also children with central, secondary CH.

-    The minimum required number of samples per laboratory was set at 30,000 per year, assuming that the high prevalence of CH in such a number would yield sufficient children with an abnormal concentration of thyroid hormone, so that loss of experience of the laboratory staff was prevented.

In the late 1980s contacts with said foreign colleagues were intensified. In previous years there was mainly written correspondence, but gradually the Dutch clinicians participated in international seminars and conferences. Thus, the LBC-CH reacted positively to an invitation from the European Society for Paediatric Endocrinology to delegate someone (Dr. M. Gons) to a European working group on CH.

Position Health Council

The screening for PKU and the pilot screening for CH were launched with ministerial approval, but without any prior advice of the Health Council. In 1975 the Minister of Health and Environmental Protection asked the Chair of the Health Council to express an opinion on the future screening package including a number of logistical issues. The Health Council established a committee which was composed of professors and lecturers in paediatrics and biochemistry, clinical chemists, a professor of cell biology and genetics, and a biologist from the RIV. An Inspector of the Ministry was an advisory member.

In 1979 the report was published (Gezondheidsraad 1979). A whole series of conditions was discussed, with particular emphasis on the prevalence, the treatability and the availability of tests. The Health Council considered conditions with a prevalence of less than 1:100,000 as being unsuitable to be included because it could lead to demotivation of the professionals involved in screening, and the costs could surpass the benefits. In addition to PKU and CH, for which there was no doubt whatsoever, only galactosemia would meet the criteria. However, the symptom-free period after birth for galactosemia is fairly short. To make a sensible screening programme, the heel prick would have to be taken earlier and that did not meet the then valid requirements for PKU screening. The prevalence of galactosemia (about 1:40,000) was deemed too low to go to much trouble to fit it into the existing system.

Start of Nationwide Programme

The first results of the pilot project on heel prick screening for hypothyroidism were so favourable (Derksen-Lubsen, 1981; GHI 1980) that, also in the light of the Health Council's report, it was decided to implement CH screening at 1 January 1981. A steering group of the Neonatal Research led by the Director-General of the RIV, Dr. H. Cohen, was concerned with the practical aspects of scaling up nationally.

In March 1980 it was finally decided that screening for CH would not only comprise the primary forms, *i.e.* with a defect in the thyroid gland, but also the central forms, with a malfunction of the pituitary gland or hypothalamus. The Netherlands thus followed the example of Canada and many states in the US, but was, and still is, an exception in Europe. The experts in other countries are of the opinion that the central forms of hypothyroidism are not serious enough to screen for. Incidentally, this is an ongoing discussion (Fisher 2005, Lanting *et al.* 2005).

Period 3: Consolidation 1981–1995

After the turbulent first years of the introduction of screening in the Netherlands for two conditions, about which there had been virtually no public discussion, a period of about 15 years followed in which the key word was 'consolidation'. Processes were streamlined, a regular meeting circuit got underway with the National Steering Committees PKU and CH as leaders. Numerous topics were discussed at length, such as the link between the screening process and the follow-up diagnostics, introduction of an annual process and effect evaluation (Meijer 1985), a progressive standardisation of processes by the various organisations involved and financing of expenses that were of interest for the programme but were not covered in the formal funding.

During this period screening was not only discussed in the 'inner circle' of paediatricians and a small group of other people involved, but gradually became known to healthcare providers, such as general practitioners and midwives, and to the general public. Such a process does not come without a struggle. Not only the advantages of the new population-wide programme but also the disadvantages were given attention, such as the finding of a false positive screening result with the consequence of a referral to the paediatrician, which afterwards proved to be unnecessary. Dealing with data files, at the time mostly handwritten, in the screening laboratories, vaccination registries, paediatricians and TNO, was settled in a privacy policy regulation document.

Evaluation and Programme of Adjustment

The annual evaluation reports of TNO showed that there were large regional differences in the rate of notification of a birth and the subsequent trajectory of heel prick sampling and sending the blood sample. Also in the process of referral to the paediatrician and follow-up diagnostics such differences in the speed of action were visible. This led to measures from the LBCs, some of them through the Inspectorate, in order to achieve better uniformity. TNO came up with suggestions to hone some screening criteria and cut off limits. This led to fewer referrals. Widening of other criteria ensured that fewer CH patients were missed, as discussed below.

CH-Screening: 'Prematures Adjustment'

As mentioned above, at the introduction of the CH-screening, it was decided on the basis of the results of the pilot region to detect both the primary and central forms of CH via a two-tiered screening. First, the concentration of thyroid hormone (T4) was determined and if it was below the cut off limit, the concentration of thyroid stimulating hormone (TSH) was determined.

A TNO study of the results of the first two years showed that this led to a much greater number of false positive referrals than expected. Premature newborns (birth weight ≤ 2500 grams and/or gestational age ≤ 36 weeks) often have relatively low levels of thyroid hormone T4, but are otherwise healthy. General practitioners and paediatricians expressed an unfavourable view of the screening programme with yet another 'wrongly' referred child. Of course all false positive results are especially difficult for the parents concerned (Tijmstra 1984). The LBC-CH decided around mid-1982 on the first amendment to the screening scheme, known as the 'prematures adjustment'. From then on the concentration of thyroid stimulating hormone TSH was the leading decision for referral of premature infants.

For this to succeed, the gestational age had to be known. However, the LBC decided this was a privacy-sensitive issue which should not be recorded for all infants on the heel prick set itself, but only if the birth weight was below 2500 grams. On the cover envelope this instruction was added. In practice, this did not work very well because not all performers read this instruction or acted accordingly. The result was that the adjustment for premature babies was not optimally implemented. With the introduction of screening for congenital adrenal hyperplasia, see below for period 4, the knowledge of gestational age would be indispensable for all newborns and recording it on the heel prick set would become an explicit instruction.

CH-Screening: Expansion with TBG

A further discussion concerning the quality of the CH-screening was related to the significance of a low-T4 concentration. Almost all T4 in the blood is bound to thyroxine-binding globulin (TBG). Therefore for a proper interpretation of the T4 concentration, the TBG concentration was also of interest.

> *The concentration of T4 may be reduced due to a low concentration of this TBG, a completely benign, genetically determined deviation. Only the unbound T4, the free T4, plays a role in the metabolism. Ideally, one would like to determine the free T4 in place of the total T4, but analytically this is complicated. To date, no one has succeeded in establishing a stable reliable method for large-scale use. Therefore, instead of measuring free T4, the attention was focused on the measuring of TBG.*

Adding a TBG determination obviously would cost extra money, so a funding source was looked for. It was decided to put the question in a research project that was honoured by the Praeventiefonds. Apart from the costs there was also the question whether in general there was enough blood on the heel prick card. The PKU-laboratories normally held two of the four spots and sent two spots to the CH-laboratories (see Chapter 2 for a description of the laboratory structure). The proposal to forward three instead of two spots initially met with some resistance in the LBC-PKU (quote from the chairman "they are our spots"), but it was agreed. The results of this pilot study proved to be very favourable. By adding a TBG assay to cards with the 5% lowest T4 concentration, the number of referrals and 2nd heel pricks (these are necessary if the screening results are not unambiguous positive or negative) on the basis of the T4/TBG-ratio were reduced by about 60%, which was a big improvement for the parents and, of course, a huge cost saving (see Figure 1.6.). On January 1, 1995, TBG determination in this manner was introduced as an integral part of the CH-screening.

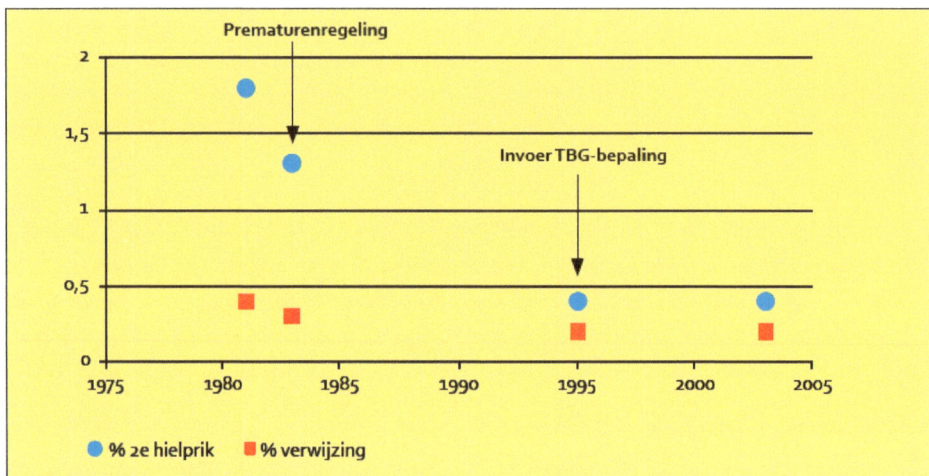

Figure 1.6. Changes in the screening system for CH and its effect on the percentage of 2nd heel pricks and referrals between 1981 and 2004 ("prematurenregeling" = premature adjustment;"invoer TBG-bepaling" = introduction of TBG-analysis; "verwijzing"=referral).

Referral and Diagnostics

The start of the neonatal screening for CH has also led to more information on the clinical diagnostics and monitoring of this heterogeneous disease. To assess whether CH in newborns is of a temporary or permanent nature, such a child should be followed intensively for several years (Vulsma 1991). In the beginning such a process of follow-up was not yet covered by the health insurance. A research project was again funded by the Praeventiefonds. The results over several years revealed that follow-up studies were inextricably linked with the screening process and the health insurers accepted to cover these costs.

At the introduction of the PKU screening it was decided that, based on the limited number of referrals per year (approximately 25), they would be done at the academic children's hospitals. At the introduction of the CH screening, however, the board of the NVK clung to the idea that because of the (much) larger number of expected referrals (300) these should be done to each paediatrician in the Netherlands. Moreover, compared to PKU, CH would be easier to treat and follow up and this could be done by a peripheral paediatrician. For parents, it would obviously be advantageous to have the treating paediatrician in close proximity. However, based on the number of paediatricians it could be calculated that on average, every paediatrician would not see a referred child more than once every 4–5 years. To assist paediatricians in the schedule of confirmatory diagnostics, the LBC-CH issued an extremely useful workbook (Figure 1.7.; Bongers *et al.* 1980.).

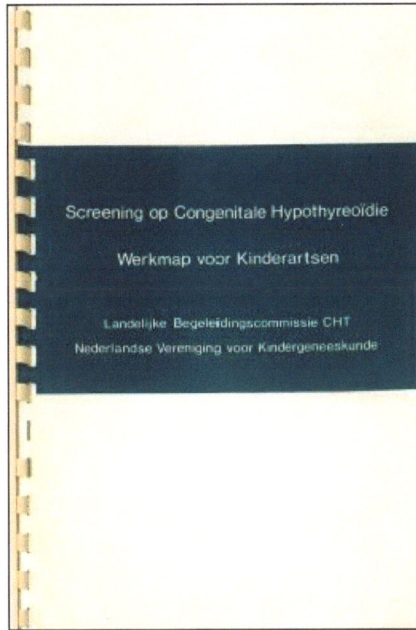

Figure 1.7. Title page of the Workbook for paediatricians to help in the diagnostics and treatment of children with abnormal CH screening results.

Unfortunately, no one had considered who would take care of the costs of printing and distribution. The LBC-CH had no resources of its own, the NVK decided that it was not its responsibility, the Inspectorate likewise, and within the financing structure of the screening programme via the AWBZ there was no provision. In the end the commercial supplier of the drug necessary for the CH patients was willing to pay the printing costs, while the NVK, albeit with great reluctance and only once, agreed to bear the cost of the shipment.

Scientific Research

In addition to performing the screening and follow-up diagnostics there arose interest in doing scientific research into the health effects achieved as a result of the screening. Eventually, of course, they wanted to know whether any efforts would lead to the desired health outcome. One of the most important studies was comparing the mental and motor development of detected PKU- and CH patients with those of healthy children (Huisman *et al*. 1985, Kalverboer and Bleeker, 1988). The main conclusion was that screening prevented intellectual disabilities, but nevertheless there were some neurological abnormalities mainly in the areas of fine and gross motor skills and body control.

Concerning PKU screening, more issues required further consideration. Many children who would have been mentally handicapped without screening could now, following a special diet, lead a fairly normal life; therefore, a good result. Initially it was thought that the diet, which was perceived as very stressful, could be discontinued in adulthood. Unfortunately, this often led to neurological symptoms recurring. The advice was therefore to continue the

19

low-protein diet for life. That was especially important in female PKU patients who were pregnant, otherwise the foetus would be exposed to high levels of phenylalanine in the mother's blood, which would lead to a delay in brain development; the so-called 'maternal PKU' (Koch *et al.*1986).

Leftover Blood Samples

The availability of the heel prick blood led to the question of whether this could be used for other research lines (Swaak 1978). For example, in 1983 the Health Council had advised to consider what the prevalence of congenital toxoplasmosis was. A research project of the RIVM to examine this in pregnant women, and subsequently in their newborns, however, was not accepted by the LBCs. An important consideration was the fear that parents could make insufficient distinction between the routine screening programme and scientific investigation and therefore probably would decline participation in the programme. After much discussion, a way was found to provide the blood spots anonymously to investigators.

Sometime later, the LBCs were asked to consider a proposal to use blood for monitoring HIV antibodies so as to get an idea of the spread of HIV in the general population. The LBCs considered this goal too distant from the goal of the screening programme and declined. Occasional requests for prevalence studies including myotonic dystrophy, Pompe disease, and long-chain fatty acid oxidation disorders were also declined. From 2000 onwards, the LBC improved the definitions of what kind of research questions the blood spots in principle could be made available for (see Chapter 2).

Discussions on Further Expansion

From the beginning of the 1990s, contacts with foreign colleagues were improved amongst others by participation in the biennial congresses in the US that were focussed on the primary screening process. In Europe, the congresses were of a much more clinical nature and the paediatric subspecialties (metabolic, endocrine) had their own individual meeting circuits, preventing a coherent picture being obtained.

During the American congresses, a recurrent topic was the ever-expanding panel of conditions eligible for screening. To arrive at a proper assessment of the advantages and disadvantages of screening for a condition, guidelines were developed. In 1975 the American Academy of Paediatrics had previously published a list of criteria (National Academy of Sciences, 1975), which had been cited in the advice of the Health Council in 1979. This list is similar to the general criteria for a responsible screening programme that Wilson and Jungner developed for the World Health Organization (Wilson and Jungner 1968).

Table 1.1. Wilson and Jungner criteria for screening (translation in Dutch RIVM 2014a).

1. The disease to be detected must be a major health problem.
2. There must be a generally accepted treatment method for the disease.
3. Satisfactory arrangements for diagnosis and treatment must be available.
4. There must be a recognizable latent or early symptomatic stage of the disease.
5. A reliable detection method must exist.
6. The detection method must be acceptable to the population.
7. The natural course of the disease being detected must be known.
8. There must be agreement on who should be treated.
9. The costs of detection, diagnosis and treatment must be in an acceptable proportion to the cost of health care as a whole.
10. The process of detection should be a continuous process and not a one-off project.

Their publication dated from 1968, *i.e.* after the screening for PKU was launched in several countries, but before the screening for CH was introduced. Around 1980, the Wilson and Jungner criteria, however, were generally accepted as a kind of gold standard in discussions about whether or not to screen for a particular condition. Over the years in the Netherlands these criteria were discussed and honed in some respects (Health Council 1989, 1994), but their general meaning was left unchanged.

In retrospect it can be said that the Dutch screening programme for PKU and CH met at least nine of the ten criteria. Criterion 9 'cost' has been mentioned in a number of Health Council Reports as a global estimate prior to an expansion of the programme (Health Council 1979, 2005, 2010). However, the real situation being practiced has in fact never been investigated in detail. A rather crude approach has been stated in the Annual Financial Review Health Care of October 1991. The figures released by the Ministry of Health indicated that the neonatal screening was extremely cost effective (De Koning *et al.* 1992).

Period 4: Congenital Adrenal Hyperplasia (CAH) 1995–2002

Based on experience abroad there was also discussion in the Netherlands whether other conditions could or should be added to the screening programme. After the Health Council Report 1979, no new inventory had been made in spite of the significant technological progress. Taking into account the above criteria of Wilson and Jungner, and building on existing analytical methods and the available equipment, congenital adrenal hyperplasia (CAH, in Dutch 'adrenogenitaal syndroom' or AGS) was the most obvious next condition after PKU and CH, though this notion was not supported by everyone.

> *In CAH the activity of one or more enzymes in the adrenal gland is so low that the conversion of cholesterol into aldosterone and cortisol is disrupted, with simultaneous accumulation of a metabolite 17α-hydroxyprogesterone and an over-production of male sex hormones. This situation can lead not only to a very severe salt loss, coma and death in the first week after birth, but also to developmental damage. In girls there is a chance that virilisation of the external genital organs that can lead to wrong gender determination, which, apart from physiological problems, of course, is traumatic for the child and the family.*

Pilot Screening

In 1987, in Nijmegen, a PhD thesis was published on CAH (Otten 1987), in which the clinical knowledge about this condition had received a base in the Netherlands. A collaboration between researchers at the Radboud UMC, TNO and RIVM was quickly forged in 1995 and a pilot project on 'Screening for CAH', after consultation with the LBCs, was submitted to the Praeventiefonds for financing. The project proposal was, albeit after some modifications, deemed fit for subsidising. However, the Praeventiefonds required that there should be prior assurances from the Ministry of Health for continuation as a regular part of the screening programme, should the results of the pilot project turned out to be favourable. That was a sort of chicken-and-egg issue because the Ministry did not want to commit itself politically, awaiting the results. After carefully formulating a sort of declaration of intent by the Ministry, the Praeventiefonds accepted the proposal for financing.

A point of discussion was whether CAH screening could be fitted into the existing programme without problems. Unlike PKU and CH, the symptomless period for CAH is just a few days after birth. Screening would only be meaningful if the age of blood sampling could be brought forward to day 5 (day of birth counted as day 0). The recommended period would thus be days 5 to day 7. Given the good results already achieved for some years with application of the Quantase method for PKU (see Section 3 for details), which was much more sensitive than the traditional Guthrie method, the LBC-PKU quickly agreed to this proposal. However, given the fact that the legal period of birth registration was three days, that then had to be followed by a signal to the person in the home health care organisation in charge of blood sampling, day 5 would hardly be feasible. It seemed that day 5 could only be realised in the provinces where the heel prick was traditionally carried out by the midwife (Gelderland and South Holland), because the midwife always does a home visit soon after birth anyway and would not have to wait on the procedure of birth registration. In practice, fortunately the results showed that even with sampling on day 5 or 6 the CAH screening result usually was available before symptoms occurred. Figure 1.8. shows how the recommended sampling period affected the percentage of children sampled on day 7 after birth.

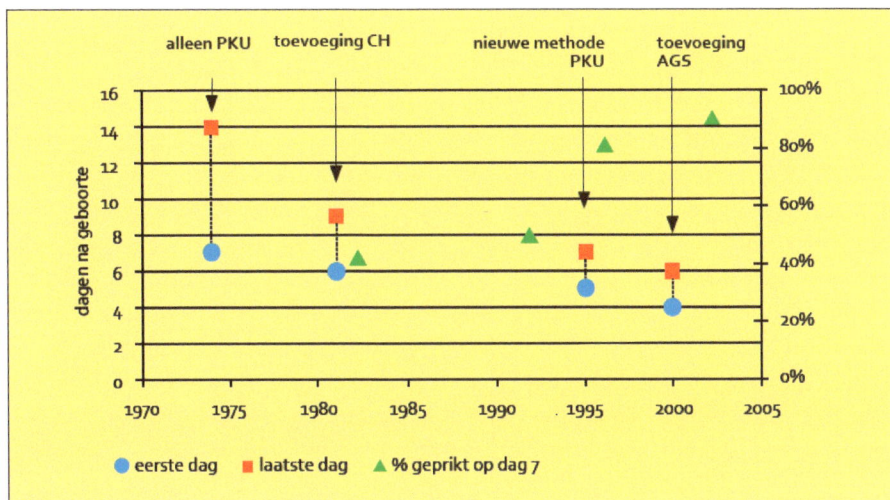

Figure 1.8. Effect of recommended sampling period on the percentage of children sampled at day 7 after birth between 1974 and 2005.("alleen"= only; "toevoeging"= addition; "AGS"= CAH).

The CAH project progressed smoothly. First, the analytical method for the steroid 17α-hydroxyprogesterone was developed on the basis of blood samples from clinically detected CAH patients, and control samples. Thus, a cut-off limit could be established. The pilot screening was set up in two of the five regions, *i.e.* the provinces of Gelderland, Utrecht, South Holland and Zeeland (see Section 2 for classification of regions). Paediatricians in the other three regions were asked to report newborns with CAH, who were detected not through screening but by clinical suspicion, to the Dutch Signalling Centre of Paediatrics (NSCK) in Leyden. Thus, a good comparison of the effectiveness of the pilot screening *versus* the existing practice was possible.

> *The NSCK was founded in 1992 by the NVK. The members of the NVK are asked to voluntarily notify the NSCK of cases of rare diseases and disorders in children of 0-18 years. After an announcement, the paediatrician receives a questionnaire for providing more detailed information. In this way data on the prevalence and spread of such diseases are collected.*

In the project group, in addition to the paediatricians, screening laboratories and TNO, now also the vaccination registries (the bodies organising the logistics for the national vaccination programme; for a description see Chapter 2) were represented to keep an eye on the practical aspects of a possible introduction. Normally the medical advisors for the vaccination registries are responsible for the referral of screen-positive children. However, it was decided that during this pilot project in the two regions, all referrals should be done by one paediatrician so that the lines with all concerned remained central and quick. The pilot project was launched on January 1, 1998. On the second day a child with CAH was detected.

Start of the Nationwide Program

Initially the project was anticipated to last for two years, after which an evaluation would follow and a decision on implementation would be taken. However, based on the favourable results of 1998 and the first half of 1999, the project group asked the Ministry in autumn 1999 for permission to continue the screening at least in the pilot regions in order to avoid interruption. This was agreed and ZonMw, successor of the Praeventiefonds, provided the financing. In 2000 and 2001 the AGS screening protocol was further refined by tightening the cut off limits. The recommended age of sampling was set to be one day earlier, *i.e.* from day 4 to day 7, with emphasis on the fact that sampling on day 4 was preferred. After the existing informative material had been expanded to include information about CAH and the preparations in the other three regions were completed, CAH was fully integrated in the neonatal screening programme from 2002 onwards (van der Kamp, 2001).

Period 5: Medium-Chain Acyl CoA Dehydrogenase Deficiency (MCADD) and Sickle Cell Disease 2002–2006

More or less simultaneously with the pilot for the CAH screening in 1998, a debate started within the LBC-PKU on the introduction of a novel technique for the detection of metabolic diseases. This technique involves the combination of two mass spectrometers, and therefore it is called tandem mass spectrometry or ms/ms.

Pilot Screening MCADD

In 2002, a proposal was launched by the Groningen University Medical Centre (UMCG) for a pilot screening on medium-chain acyl CoA dehydrogenase deficiency (MCADD), a disorder of fatty acid degradation.

> *Medium-chain acyl CoA dehydrogenase is an enzyme involved in the metabolism of fatty acids from food, producing energy. Its deficiency (MCADD) causes a shortage of energy, which can lead to sudden coma or infant death when the child has an acute energy need. Such situations can be prevented by frequent feeding of smaller portions. In Groningen, in 1994-1995 an anonymous prevalence study had been conducted (De Vries et al. 1996). The results indicated that in the Netherlands the prevalence was high enough to consider screening.*

MCADD can only be detected via tandem mass spectrometry (see Chapter 3). At that moment the costly equipment was only available for diagnostic purposes in university medical centres. The pilot screening, funded by ZonMw, started in the northern region of the country (the provinces of Groningen, Friesland, Drenthe and Overijssel) in the spring of 2003. After finishing the 'regular' screening, the laboratory in the city of Zwolle sent the heel prick cards to UMCG for the MCADD analysis. Just as in the case of the pilot screening for CAH, the referrals were not done by the medical advisors of the vaccination registries, but by paediatricians temporarily employed by UMCG.

The project went well and the number of referred children was as expected (Derks 2007). In principle the project was to run until the end of 2005, after which a decision would be taken on whether MCADD would be added to the screening panel. The decision, however, was overtaken by the establishment of a new Health Council Committee (see below, 'Period 6').

Pilot Screening Sickle Cell Disease

In parallel, sickle cell anaemia came on the agenda. This disorder is rarely present in people that originate from Northern European countries. As a consequence of increased migration after World War II by persons originating from countries in Africa, the Mediterranean or Asia, the prevalence of sickle cell anaemia in the Netherlands had risen to such a level that screening was considered. Though in theory only infants from originally non-northern-European ancestry would qualify for screening, in practice it would be really difficult to establish the precise ethnicity of a baby. Therefore it was decided to screen all newborns. In 2003, ZonMw decided to fund a pilot of the university medical centres, AMC, VUmc, LUMC, as well as RIVM, led by TNO. In the middle region (provinces of Utrecht and Gelderland) and south-west region (provinces of Zuid Holland and Zeeland) newborns were screened for sickle cell anaemia. When a positive result was obtained, the card was sent to the reference laboratory for sickle cell anaemia in the LUMC for confirmation and characterisation. The other project partners covered societal aspects of a potential implementation. The results of this pilot were used by the new Health Council Committee for its upcoming advice (see below, 'Period 6').

Period 6: An Extended Screening Panel 2003–2007

New Techniques and Their Consequences

Tandem mass spectrometry allowed for extension of the number of disorders in the heel prick programme. The LBC-PKU saw big advantages, but also drawbacks because by using this technique, information can be obtained relatively easily about diseases for which no treatment is available. In this way points 2 and 3 of Wilson and Jungner's criteria could no longer be met. In short: ethical dilemmas. Given the uncertain status of the LBCs at that time and the then ongoing discussion about the transfer of the programme to the Ziekenfondsraad/CVZ (see Chapter 2) it did not seem wise for them to take such a decision.

In 2002 a workshop was organised by the Health Council in collaboration with ZonMw on the implications of using tandem mass spectrometry and, in 2001, an ethical 'Signalling study' was published (Gezondheidsraad 2003a,b). It discussed especially challenges in relation to the number and kind of conditions to be screened for, and the consequences concerning parents' informed choice.

Health Council Committee on Neonatal Screening

By the end of 2003, at the request of the Minister, the Health Council appointed a committee on Neonatal Screening to report on how the screening programme could be extended. Reasons given were developments in detecting and treating disorders and the changing composition of the population. The composition of the committee was somewhat more diverse than in 1979. In addition to paediatricians, a biochemist, clinical chemist and clinical geneticist, now also a professor in community genetics, an ethicist, a gynaecologist and a health law professor formed part of the committee, and, as before, an advisor from the Ministry attended. The advice was published in the summer of 2005 (Gezondheidsraad 2005). The committee examined about 30 disorders and evaluated medical severity, treatability, and available screening methods, and came to a trichotomy.

> The Health Council committee discerned three categories of disorders: disorders for which considerable, irreversible health damage could be prevented if detected in time (category 1), disorders for which that was less the case or for which insufficient evidence could be established (category 2), and disorders for which no health damage could be prevented by neonatal screening.
>
> The Health Council committee also focused on carrier status and how to deal with information regarding carrier status. Finding an affected child automatically implies that both parents must be carriers for that disorder. The parents themselves are not affected but carry a mutation on one of the two alleles of the gene involved in that disorder. Another finding from the screening might be that the child is not affected but is a carrier him- or herself. In that case at least one of the parents must also be a carrier for that disorder. For the parents, carrier status information is important because subsequent children may also be affected if both parents are carriers. This

aspect was not new, as already at the preparation of the screening programme in 1970 the possibility to find carriers had been recognized (Study Group Phenylketonuria 1970). The question arose how to deal with this information. The child cannot decide for him- or herself whether he or she would want to have this information on carrier status. The 'right not to know' of a child would be compromised. In the early years the available options were not having (any more) children or finding another partner; later technological developments made it possible for some disorders to opt for prenatal screening in a subsequent pregnancy, seeking donors for sperm or oocytes, or having pre implantation genetic diagnosis.

The Health Council committee discussed at length how to deal with screening for untreatable disorders (category 3, above); a subject that has been on the agenda for many years. Already in 1979 the Health Council indicated that though this was not within its remit, it was important to start public debate on this topic in a timely manner. Over the years arguments regarding pro and con screening for untreatable disorders were discussed. A relevant question in this respect is whether screening is primarily in the child's best interest or also in the interest of the parents. The possibility to enable parents having reproductive choices is an important argument, especially in case of untreatable disorders. However, this might also be in the child's best interest. If several affected children would be born in one family, the first affected child may receive less care and attention (De Wert 2005). A long diagnostic trajectory can be avoided in which parents are very concerned about health problems and the child is subjected to all kind of medical examinations. Parents may support their child better and from an early stage, extra attention and care may help keep the child in relatively good condition. Also scientific research is possible to study the effect of treatments and supportive measures. The notion of 'treatment' has evolved. Disorders might not be completely curable, but sometimes supportive measures may result in considerable improvement. Disadvantages are that parents may be deprived of the first happy period with their child, it is a heavy burden knowing the child is seriously ill or will fall ill without there being much that can be done. Problems in the attachment between parents and child may occur, and also the child him- or herself has been unable to decide regarding receiving relevant health information.

For the committee, health gain for the child as a direct benefit of screening was central. In addition, screening might have indirect benefits for the child, such as improvement of diagnostics or care. When screening would not lead to the prevention of health damage, as in the case of untreatable disorders, it was decided not to screen for such a disorder. In this way the Health Council kept and acknowledged the framework for screening as was established at the start of screening. On this basis it was proposed to add 15 disorders to the screening panel.

Table 1.2. Additional Disorders to Be Screened for after 2007.

Biotinidase deficiency
Cystic fibrosis (conditionally)
Galactosemia
Glutaric aciduria type I
HMG-CoA lyase (3-hydroxy-3-methylglutaric acid-CoA-lyase) deficiency
Holocarboxylase synthase deficiency
Homocystinuria
Isovaleric acidemia
Long-chain hydroxyacyl-CoA dehydrogenase deficiency
Maple syrup urine disease
Medium-chain Acyl-CoA dehydrogenase deficiency
3-Methylcrotonyl-CoA carboxylase deficiency
Sickle cell disease
Tyrosinemia
Very long-chain acyl-CoA dehydrogenase deficiency

In the case of cystic fibrosis (CF) it was evident that screening led to health gain: fewer hospital admissions would be needed and nutritional status would be better. However, there were doubts about the test, most notably its specificity, which might lead to a high number of false positive results. It was advised to integrate CF in the screening panel on the condition that a better test would become available. Also the indirect advantages for the child or the family were brought to attention. Neonatal screening would prevent a long diagnostic quest. Because of the hereditary nature of the disorder (as most disorders in the heel prick programme) parents would be informed in time on the risks related to a subsequent pregnancy, so they could make an informed reproductive choice.

The advice was well received at the Ministry. By late November 2005, the Ministry decided to follow the advice and set the date for expansion of the programme at 1 January 2007.

Preparations on Many Domains

The year 2006 was perhaps the most turbulent one of the whole described period of 40 years. Previous expansions of the screening panel consisted of adding one disease at a time, now 14 disorders were involved, including 13 metabolic diseases, and sickle cell disease.

Establishing the Centre for Population Screening

On January 1, 2006, the RIVM established a new centre, the Centre for Population Screening (CvB). Its main task was to coordinate the national screening programmes, including the neonatal programme, on behalf of the Ministry. This implied that after several decades, the government itself became involved in managing the daily affairs of the neonatal screening programme. For the CvB this meant that from the first day on, not only a new organisation had to be established, but also the neonatal screening programme had to be urgently taken up. The CvB established a programme committee for Neonatal Heel Prick Screening with representatives of the various professional groups and organisations involved with the screening. For more details, see Chapter 2.

Screening Laboratories

The screening laboratories were instructed to quickly start preparations for the purchase and use of tandem mass spectrometers, equipment that was relatively unknown to these laboratories (see Chapter 3). The metabolic centres in the university hospitals that did have this knowledge and experience argued for the screening to be performed by themselves. A big drawback would have been that for the different groups of disorders, different routes for sending heel prick blood samples would have to be established, or that in the recipient laboratory the blood samples would have to be separated and forwarded on; a situation that had just been ended in 1995 (see Chapter 2).

After the choice for a supplier of this equipment had been made, detailed instruction sessions for laboratory staff and employees followed. Subsequently, analytical cut-off levels had to be established for each disorder. For this, good use was made of the experience of the above-mentioned MCADD project in Groningen and information from foreign colleagues.

Sickle cell disease required yet another method of analysis, namely high pressure liquid chromatography (see Chapter 3). Here the choice of the type of instrument was much more difficult. A pilot with tens of thousands of samples in two laboratories led to the final choice, after which the employees had to be trained for working with that equipment as well.

Information Materials

To develop information material for parents and screeners, the CvB set up a working group 'Expertise Promotion' with representatives of the various disciplines. The administrative systems at the vaccination registries were adapted to accommodate the larger number of disorders and their results, and were aligned with the systems of the screening laboratories. Increasingly, communication between laboratories and vaccination registries became electronic.

Diagnostics

For the academic children's clinics, the problem was slightly different. Their knowledge about the new conditions was sufficient, but they feared a large increase in referred children that would turn out not to be ill: the false positives that occur in each extension of a screening programme. The metabolic paediatricians of each children's clinic insisted on funding for expansion of capacity for personnel, but it was unclear who could make such a decision. This was an example of the segregation in Dutch healthcare between public health care and curative health care. The Minister deals with the screening process in the strict sense, *i.e.* up to the referral of the children identified through screening, but has no direct control over the follow-up. The confirmation of the diagnosis and possible treatment is the domain of medical professionals and health care insurers. However, it is clear that screening and diagnostics are inextricably linked and that data from both trajectories should be brought together to enable monitoring and optimisation of the system.

The CvB that had yet to establish its position, was faced with the above mentioned dilemma. The difficult relationship between the Ministry, CvB, the paediatrician's society NVK and other parties gradually developed in a positive manner. The much lower than expected number of false positives was a pleasant piece of good luck. In this way, CvB managed to bring the parties together in 2009 and persuaded them to adopt a practical mode of operation. The requested additional funding was never realised. Especially paediatricians still regularly draw attention to the fact that there is hardly any budget for additional follow-up examinations, with the exception of some disorder-specific budgets funded by ZonMw.

Starting up in 2007

The hard work done in 2006 was rewarded. The extended screening programme was indeed running from 2007. In practice, however, 2007 was a kind of pilot year in which still a few practical issues needed to be resolved despite the good preparation. The large number of false-positive galactosemia referrals was remarkable and other determinations and cut off limits had to be established. The method chosen for tyrosinemia type 1 was found not to be adequate, this part was suspended for over a year until the vendor was able to supply improved reagents. These setbacks prompted a critical article in *Medisch Contact* (Niermeijer *et al.* 2007).

Much discussion focused on sickle cell screening and especially on the sickle cell carriers. As indicated above, carriers have one gene variant that is related to the disorder in combination with one healthy gene variant. The latter one dominates and the person does not become ill. A screening programme is generally not focused on identifying carriers, on the contrary, in accordance with the aim of screening, one tries not to detect them. However, the screening method chosen for sickle cell disease also detected a large number of carriers. Unfortunately, no other suitable methods were available. The dilemma was how to deal with this information. The information flyer tried to explain the matter as well as possible. At the time of the heel prick, the parents were able to indicate whether they wanted to receive the carrier status information or not. In practice, only a few parents objected to receiving this information. From an evaluation study it appeared that parents often did not realise that the carrier status information was relevant for themselves in relation to a subsequent pregnancy (Van der Pal et al. 2010).

Besides sickle cell carriers also children with beta thalassemia major and alpha thalassemia were detected. In its 2005 Advice, the Health Council had treated thalassemia as a category 2 disease, a view that was not shared by all paediatric haematologists. Since it appeared now that the children in question could be identified without much difficulty, an agreement was reached on clinical relevance and treatability of thalassemia, and after some months of discussion, thalassemia was also reported.

The results of the extended screening for 2007 and 2008 were published in four articles (Visser et al. 2009; Peters et al. 2009; Vansenne et al. 2009; Kemper -Proper et al. 2009). In addition, the results were part of the annual reporting by TNO (Verkerk *et al*. 1991–2012).

Period 7: Cystic Fibrosis (CF) 2007–2011

In the 2005 Advice of the Health Council, screening for cystic fibrosis (CF) was recommended, provided that a better method became available.

> *Cystic Fibrosis, is a disorder in which several organs, e.g. the lungs and the gastrointestinal tract, the mucus is sticky. In the respiratory tract accumulation of mucus occurs that can lead to chronic infections and damage to the lungs. In the pancreas, clogging of the drainage channels leads to a reduction of digestive enzymes in the intestine. Impaired absorption of nutrients causes fatty diarrhea, malnutrition and growth retardation. The sweat of CF patients contains more salt, which can be demonstrated via the so-called sweat test.*

A project proposal to find out how to improve the method of analysis was paid for by ZonMw. It was called CHOPIN (Cystic fibrosis Heel Prick research In Newborns In the Netherlands) Preparations started in 2007 with the intention to perform a pilot screening in four provinces (Gelderland, Utrecht, Noord Brabant and Limburg) in 2008 and 2009.

In the literature, two screening variants were central. In the first, the concentration of two different proteins was measured and, in case of an abnormal result, the newborn would be subjected to a so-called sweat test, in which the sweat was checked for the level of salt. In the second, the concentration of one of the proteins was measured and, in case of an abnormal result, the same blood sample would be tested for a range of DNA mutations. If certain mutations occurred, again a sweat test was performed.

In this pilot screening the two variants were compared by running them in parallel for all heel prick blood samples. After detailed analysis of all data, a combination of the two variants proved to be optimal (Vernooij-van Langen, 2013).

> *Thus for CF, a four-tiered screening model resulted in which first the concentration of immunoreactive trypsinogen is determined (Step 1). If this is above the cut-off limit, then the concentration of pancreatitis-associated protein is determined (Step 2). If this marker is also above the threshold, a limited DNA mutation analysis is performed for which a panel of the 36 most common mutations is used (Step 3). If two mutations are detected, the child is referred further, and if only one mutation is found, then the DNA is sequenced (Step 4). If that leads to a second mutation, then the child is also referred further. This extra step is important because the 36 mutations from the panel are mostly present in parents who originally come from northern Europe, whereas some migrant groups from, e.g. Turkey have other, partly unknown, CF-mutations. The result of this fairly complex procedure is that few carriers are found and only a small number of false positives occur, and that the changing composition of the population can be taken into account.*

In principle, the Ministry was positive about adding CF to the screening panel but wanted to have the opinion from the Health Council first. Some of the previous members of the Neonatal Screening committee from 2005 were installed again in a new committee in 2010, and a positive advice quickly followed (Gezondheidsraad 2010). As of May 1, 2011, CF was part of the screening panel.

Period 8: Future Expansions in 2011 and Beyond

Technical developments never stop. Continually, new conditions are described in the literature as suitable candidates to be included in the panel. Each time the question arises whether such a situation would meet the Wilson and Jungner criteria. Especially the aspect of (un)treatability is an important issue. Here a contrast emerges between the cautious approach of the government focusing on the benefit for the screened child and concentrating on health gain, and the opinion of (some of the) parents ("the more I know about my child, the better, then I am already prepared for illness, and I can take this into account also in case of a future pregnancy" (Tijmstra *et al.* 2008).

In January 2013, the next Health Council Committee on Neonatal Screening was installed with the mission to advise on lysosomal storage disorders (Pompe, Krabbe, Gaucher, *etc.*), severe combined immunodeficiency (SCID) and Duchenne muscular dystrophy. The report was published in 2015; and developments will continue, there are still dozens of disorders to be assessed. For most, no effective treatment is possible, but that could change quickly if, for instance, stem cell transplantation works out, such as became apparent in the case of SCID.

Screening in the Dutch Caribbean

Another development in recent years is the implementation of neonatal screening in the Dutch Caribbean (CN) and potentially also in/on other islands of the former Netherlands Antilles. However, this is not entirely new, as there have been contacts already 20 years ago. For instance, in 1994 a request was made by a general practitioner in Aruba to screen children in accordance with the Dutch system. Simple question, but difficult to answer. At that time, Aruba was already part of the Kingdom of the Netherlands but with a separate status and its own government. The Ministry in the Netherlands did not respond enthusiastically as the general policy was that Aruba itself had chosen for an independent status, with all its consequences.

Although over the years a small flow of samples was sent, until now no formal arrangement has been established. Also a paediatrician from St. Maarten has sent blood samples from time to time since the 1990s. No appropriate procedures had been agreed upon, neither for logistics, nor for (medical) responsibility, and this was not only the case for samples from the Antilles, but also for samples from other countries. The LBCs decided that such requests should be dealt with by the vaccination registry and medical advisor in the province of Utrecht and that the heel prick samples would be analysed by RIVM.

In October 2012 the Antilles were dissolved as a separate political entity and the islands Bonaire, Saint Eustace and Saba became special municipalities of the Netherlands. The inhabitants received rights and duties comparable to those of inhabitants of the Netherlands, also in health care, most notably in relation to infectious diseases (vaccinations, *etc.*).

At the same time, the subject of heel prick screening surfaced on the agenda. The CvB met with representatives of the authorities in CN to see how to set up screening logistically. Of course there were many questions. How should parents be informed, what would the screening panel look like, how should the heel prick be done, how to deal with referrals to the paediatrician?

It was clear that sickle cell would be part of the package, but for the other disorders in the 'Dutch' panel, no data were available on prevalence—the extent to which a disease occurs. Given the small number of births, from the beginning it was evident that the laboratory analyses would not be performed in CN but in the Netherlands. Logistically the easiest way would be to use the Dutch panel. Referral of newborns would be dependent on the disease. Sickle cell disease would be treated locally while other diseases would be treated partly locally and partly in the Netherlands.

Another practical complication was the fact that pregnant women from Saint Eustace and Saba nearly all go to nearby Saint Martin to give birth and stay there for several days. The heel prick has to be done by health care workers from Saint Martin, that is not part of CN itself—and while newborns from Saint Eustace and Saba are entitled to get the heel prick screening, those from Saint Martin are not. All these issues are the subject of a feasibility study carried out by the CvB (Figure 1.9.).

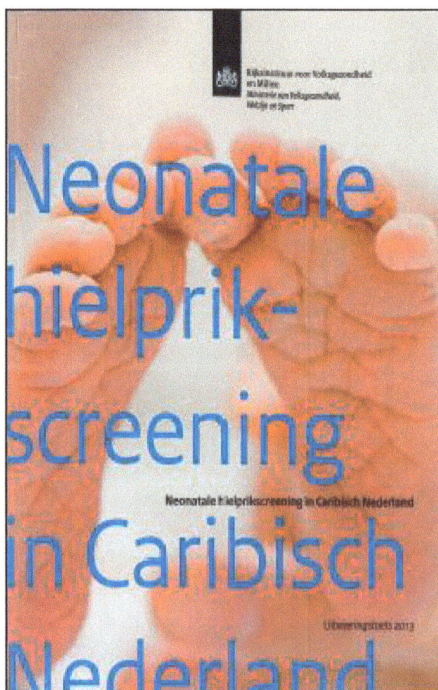

Figure 1.9. Title page of the 'Feasibility study' screening in the Dutch Caribbean.

The result is that in the beginning of 2015, screening will start in Bonaire, after which in 2015 or 2016 also Saint Eustace and Saba will join. Also Saint Martin has formally indicated that it would like to participate. Possibly Curacao and Aruba may join later.

Chapter 2: Organisational Aspects, Windfalls and Setbacks

National Consultations over the Years

From the beginning of the screening programme, the National Advisory PKU (LBC-PKU) acted as the policy oriented organisation. When the CH screening started, a separate LBC was created including a number of members of the "LBC-PKU for the necessary horizontal alignment. Due to the low prevalence of PKU and the complicated diagnostics and treatment, at the start of the screening it had been agreed that children with an abnormal screening result would be referred to one of the academic children's hospitals. As a result, the LBC-PKU was predominantly clinically oriented and consisted largely of academic active metabolic paediatricians. During the semi-annual meetings part of the time was devoted to the discussion of individual patients.

For CH, in contrast, under pressure from the NVK it was agreed that referral would be made to all paediatricians in the Netherlands. Therefore, there was less opportunity for a central discussion of patients and patient management. However, there was a need for a central protocol for follow-up diagnosis and treatment. The NVK, on the advice of the LBC-CH, implemented a separate National Advisory Committee CH (LAC-CH). Due to the fact that the CH-screening was subject to a number of organisational changes, the LBC-CH focused more and more on the monitoring of the whole screening process. The necessary coordination with the LBC-PKU was established via a small number of individuals who were part of both LBCs such as the representatives of the Health Care Inspectorate, the provincial paediatricians/medical consultants, the RIVM and TNO. The two LBCs met consecutively. This led to the situation where some topics came twice to the table, which of course was not very efficient.

In 1995 this led to the proposal to establish an overarching screening steering committee that was to be supported by the LAC-CH and a (yet to be established) LAC-PKU to advise concerning the clinical aspects. Meanwhile in 1993 the RIVM had passed the governance of the national *prenatal* screening programmes to the so called Ziekenfondsraad ('Insurance Council'), who had instituted a Pre- and Postnatal Screening Commission (CPPS). It seemed logical to position the proposed steering committee plus the LACs in some way under the CPPS. A difficult point was that the LBCs and the LACs had been established by the NVK, which was afraid to lose influence by giving up these committees.

Further delay was caused by the elimination of the Ziekenfondsraad in 1999 and the transition of its department that was involved in the screening to the Health Care Insurance Board (CVZ), one of the two parts in which the Ziekenfondsraad was split. In the meantime the LBCs had decided to restructure their consecutive meetings such that there was a joint period to discuss the common issues. Eventually the aforementioned steering committee was established by CVZ in 2003—*i.e.*, eight years after the first initiative—as the National Advisory Committee for Neonatal Screening (LBNS). The LBCs PKU and CH were disbanded by April 1, 2003.

Nonetheless, CVZ did not really know how to position the LBNS in terms of responsibility and accountability. The organisation commissioned a study by NIVEL (van der Putten *et al.*, 2005). The conclusion was that the screening programme in practice was supported by a very small number of people involved in the provincial vaccination registries and the RIVM, which was assessed as a vulnerable situation. However, before this report could lead to organisational changes within CVZ, the Centre for Population Research (CvB) was established within the RIVM on 1 January 2006.

The CvB management was given the task to steer the national screening programmes on behalf of the Ministry, including the neonatal programme. The CvB management established a Neonatal newborn blood spot screening Programme committee (PNHS), as successor to the LBNS which had functioned within CVZ since 2003. Within the PNHS again all professional groups and organisational bodies involved in the screening programme were brought together. A new element was that representatives of parents and patients were now included. The aforementioned National Advisory Committees of the NVK (LACs) were renamed Neonatal newborn blood spot screening advisory committees (ANHSs). There is an ANHS for each group of screened diseases; currently five. The Advisory Committees focus specifically on the diagnostic process after referral on the basis of the screening results. They have a representative in the PNHS thus facilitating control of the whole screening chain. The PNHS is supported by a number of working groups. The whole structure is shown in Figure 2.1.

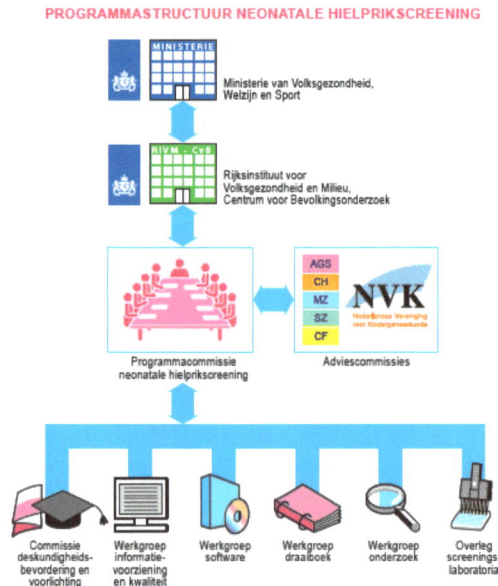

Figure 2.1. Organisation of the screening programme in 2014.

Organisation of the Vaccination Registries over the Years

At the beginning of the screening programme, it was decided that the provincial health care associations were responsible for the registration of the screening results. They already had a record of all newborn children aiming to implement the National Immunisation Programme. This component was called the provincial Vaccination Registry. All provinces and the municipalities of Amsterdam and Rotterdam had their own Vaccination Registry (Figure 2.2. a).

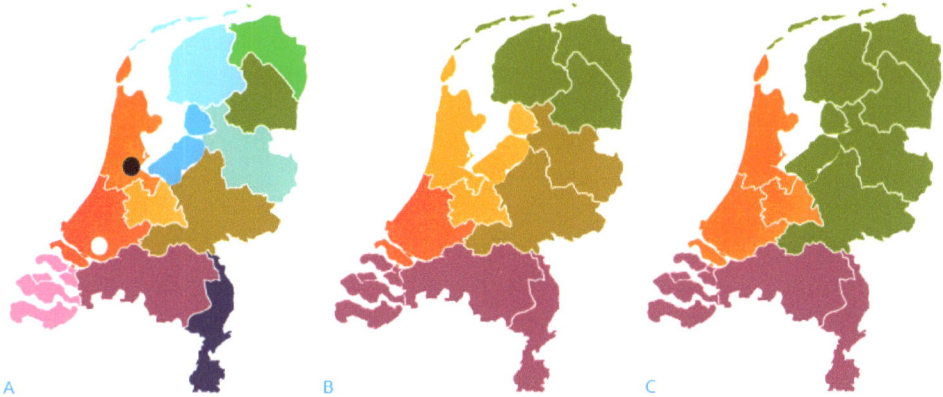

Figure 2.2. Organisation of the vaccination registries. (**a**) Situation from 1974–2008; registries in each province plus Amsterdam and Rotterdam; (**b**) Situation 2008–2013 merging into five regional offices; (**c**) Situation from 2014 further consolidation into three regional offices.

The provincial health care associations were abolished in the 1990s, whereas the vaccination registries remained. In some provinces the registries continued independently, e.g. as a foundation, in other provinces they were part of a health care organisation.

Establishment of the LVE

In the late 1990s, there were 13 vaccination registries consisting of 11 autonomous foundations and two metropolitan entities as part of the municipal health office (Amsterdam and Rotterdam). Each registry employed a medical consultant, *i.e.* the former Provincial Youth Health Care medical doctors.

In the early years, the registries received the birth notification by surface mail from the Population Division of each municipality. The laboratory results also arrived by surface mail and had to be manually linked to the child data. Consequently, there was every reason to work towards some form of automation. The group of 13 registries was divided into three groups, one of nine registries, one of three registries and a single registry. Each group developed its own IT infrastructure.

The National Association for Home Care (LVT) acted as coordinator of the vaccination registries but had no decision-making powers; every vaccination registry was autonomous in its decisions. It is clear that this did not contribute to overall efficiency, e.g. when connecting to the laboratory IT-structure or in reports to TNO.

By the end of 1997, the National Association of Vaccination Registries (Landelijke Vereniging van Entadministraties, LVE) was established, in which all vaccination registries joined. In order to increase efficiency it was decided to decrease the number of registries by merging them first to nine, later to five registries. Together they decided, under the aegis of the LVE, to build a common IT-system in combination with a national neonatal screening database. In the summer of 2005, this system was started and named Praeventis.

From LVE to RIVM

In 2005 the RIVM Centre for Infectious Disease Control was established, with the aim to restructure and harmonise the tasks in the field of public health and infectious diseases. An important element was the national vaccination programme. The Director of the Centre for Infectious Disease Control realised that he had no decision-making powers over the vaccination registries which are essential for the daily management of the National Vaccination Programme. Therefore he wanted to bring that task within the RIVM. When it became clear that the vaccination registries did not agree because this would lead to an inefficient fragmenting of their staffing, it was then decided to bring the registries in their entirety from 2008 onwards organisationally within the RIVM. The five regional registries remained physically in the periphery to allow an efficient distribution network for vaccine supply.

With this integration into the RIVM the regional registries became part of the Centre for Infectious Disease Control under the name of Regional Coordination Programmes (RCP), see Figure 2.2. b. After several reorganisations the registries on January 1, 2014 became part of the RIVM Unit Vaccine Provision and Prevention Programmes (DVP). Furthermore, it has now been decided to reduce the number of regional registries by 2015 to three in total, see Figure 2.2. c.

Organisation of the Screening Laboratories over the Years

Network of Regional Laboratories for PKU screening

Since the beginning of the screening programme in the 1960s there have been many changes in the infrastructure of the screening laboratories. One of the tasks of the RIV was to monitor the presence and emergence of infectious diseases and it needed data from across the country. To simplify the sample shipment for infectious disease diagnosis, a network of regional microbiological laboratories, partly independently, partly housed in a hospital, was established. These 18 (later 16) laboratories were called Regional Laboratories for Public Health.

When the pilot screening for PKU was planned to start in 1967 in the northern Netherlands, suitable laboratories had to be found. Given the microbiological nature of the chosen method (the Guthrie bacterial inhibition assay) it was not illogical that the RIV preferred two laboratories in this network of Regional Laboratories for Public Health.

Then, when subsequently nationwide PKU screening was implemented in 1974, it was self-evident to involve the rest of the network.

The introduction of the PKU screening was not without organisational troubles. For example, the work of the provincial health care associations, who were responsible for the registration and referrals, was organized per province whereas the 16 Regional Laboratories for Public Health served areas across province borders. A Regional Laboratory could therefore have to deal with multiple provincial health care associations and *vice versa*. The province of Gelderland had to interact with five Regional Laboratories. There were a total of 29 (!) combinations of reporting lines between Regional Labs and provincial health care organisations; in short an administrative disaster (Figure 2.3a).

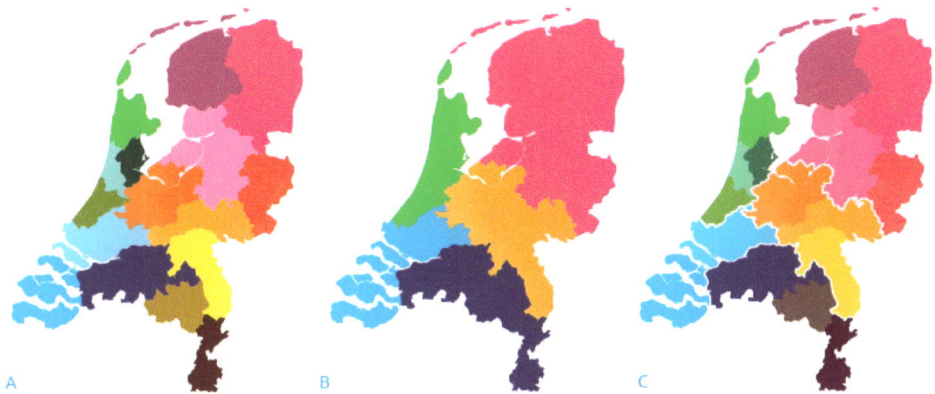

Figure 2.3. Organisation of the screening laboratories. (**a**) Network of 16 PKU-laboratories from 1974–1986; (**b**) Network of five CH-laboratories from 1981–1986; (**c**) Regional cooperation between PKU- and CH-laboratories 1981–1986.

Network of Clinical Chemical Laboratories for CH Screening

As previously indicated, the screening for CH was carried out using (radio)immunochemical methods. The methodological knowledge and equipment required was in the field of clinical chemistry laboratories and it was impossible for the screening programme to use the network of the microbiological Regional Labs. Furthermore, it was necessary for statistical reasons, to keep the number of samples per day sufficient in size and the number of laboratories, therefore, to be limited to a maximum of five. That necessitated a second network (Figure 2.3. b). Therefore, at the start of the CH-screening there were 18 Regional Laboratories for the PKU screening, four clinical chemistry laboratories for the CH-screening, whereas, within the RIV, one laboratory performed both the PKU- and the CH-screening. It was further decided that the blood spot samples initially would be sent to the PKU-laboratories which would then transmit two of the four blood spots to the CH-laboratory in the respective area of adherence (Figure 2.3. c).

41

Bundling into Five Regions

It soon became clear how much administrative burden the chosen structure of laboratories entailed. For the vaccination registries it was a hassle to get the results from two sides for all children and to check for completeness. Furthermore the forwarding by surface mail by the PKU-laboratory of the two blood spots to the CH-laboratory obviously meant a delay while sometimes a shipment by mail was lost altogether, and children had to be resampled. In 1982, the first discussions started about a simplification that eventually was completed by January 1, 1986. On that date, the number of Regional Laboratories where the PKU-screening was carried out, was reduced from 16 to five, with a simultaneous change of the working area of the screening laboratories. Five geographic regions were chosen whose boundaries coincided with provincial boundaries, with each region having one PKU-laboratory and one CH-laboratory (Figure 2.3. a). In the region 'Central' encompassing the provinces of Gelderland and Utrecht, the RIVM acted as a laboratory for both PKU and CH.

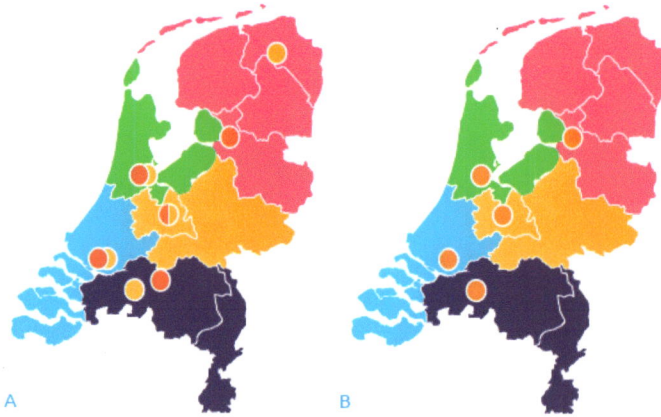

Figure 2.4. Gradual merge of laboratory networks. (**A**) Five regions, each with a PKU- and a CH-laboratory from 1986–1995; (**B**) Combined PKU/CH-laboratories 1995–present.

Such a decision sounds simple, but has in practice caused all kinds of problems. The regions had to be large enough that per laboratory a sufficient number (more than 30,000) neonatal blood samples per year would be available; the laboratories that would lose the business had to be compensated; the screening process in those laboratories obviously could not be interrupted so the blood samples had to be sent to these laboratories until the very end of 1985 and from the beginning of 1986 to other laboratories. This required care when shipping samples by those who took the blood sample. Also the heel prick test kits had to be exchanged in time with new ones with a postal code that corresponded to the new regions.

Merging the PKU- and CH-Laboratories

The next major change took place by January 1, 1995. The RIVM had already decided in 1992 that from that date the PKU screening would be performed by the CH-laboratories. The RIVM itself had combined both types of laboratory activities since the beginning of the

CH screening. The main reasons for the merger were: (1) The shortening of the turn over time of CH-screening, because there was no longer the need to split and transmit a portion of the blood sample; and (2) cost savings because the administrative burden was reduced and further automation simplified with a smaller number of parties involved. The availability of a commercial colorimetric method for the determination of phenylalanine (Elvers *et al*.1995), replacing the bacterial inhibition test, caused the heads of the microbiological Regional Labs to agree, albeit with understandable reluctance. Logistical changes were, compared with the situation at the beginning of 1986 (see above), now much simpler. The only change was the necessity to change the address on the envelopes for sending the blood sample after collection (Figure 2.3. b).

This structure of four clinical chemical screening laboratories plus the RIVM reference laboratory has worked well to date. The ever expanding screening package made frequent consultations necessary, sometimes almost daily. A group of five is large enough to conduct scientific discussions about the best approach to new developments, but also small enough to be able to come to quick decisions.

Role of the RIVM Laboratory

Of course there were questions about the fact that the RIVM was not only designated as the reference laboratory (see Chapter 1), but also was one of the screening laboratories. Would there not be a conflict of interest? However, it was soon clear that within the screening laboratories every day, so many technical and logistical issues occur that a reference laboratory cannot function as such if it is not involved in the daily operations. In all reports concerning the laboratories they were and are identified by name so that the reference laboratory with respect to its performance can be judged in the same way as the other laboratories.

A similar debate arose in 2006 with the establishment of the Centre for Population Research within the RIVM. Was it desirable that the RIVM had become the manager of the entire programme, while the reference laboratory and from 2008 onwards also the vaccination registries were part of the RIVM? By positioning these different entities in different divisions, the RIVM has tried to make clear that they are independent operating units. In addition, there is an annual process and impact evaluation by an external institution, *i.e.* TNO.

Annual Evaluation of the Program; Privacy Issues

TNO's Evaluation Role

With a population-wide screening programme, many groups and individuals are involved. There is a huge amount of personal data. Although attempts were made to register minimal personal information of the newborns, such information is often necessary for unambiguous identification of a child; for example, if it should be referred to a paediatrician. The effectiveness of the programme can best be assessed by an annual review. From the very beginning this was carried out by TNO, based on data provided by the vaccination registries, screening laboratories and the paediatricians involved. The latter group rightfully argued that a privacy regulation had to be developed in order to set clear responsibilities for these data.

The development of such a regulation by TNO and representatives of the paediatricians proved a difficult task: the first draft was already adopted in 1990; the final version not before 1996.

The evaluation focused on the children who were referred to a paediatrician, based on the screening results. For these children, the screening result was obtained from the vaccination registries/RCP and included the name of the attending paediatrician. The paediatrician was then asked to complete a form on the confirmatory diagnostics and treatment. The data could also show how long the intervals were between birth and heel prick, between heel prick and analysis, the duration of the referral process, and the age of the child at the first treatment. The annual results (Verkerk *et al.* 1991–2012) showed important regional differences in these intervals that were caused by local or regional practices and agreements between professional groups. Because of these differences, steps were taken, through many and sometimes difficult briefings to the relevant professionals, to clarify how time-critical neonatal screening is for the child in question and that each day of delay may have direct consequences for its health and development.

From Paper to Database

In the early years, data were collected via paper forms that had to be completed and then sent by surface mail. In particular, diagnostics data from paediatricians were often incomplete because of lack of time. TNO, like the vaccination registries/RCP and the screening laboratories, spent a lot of effort in the automation of the data collection which could detect much faster which data were missing and why.

Ownership of the data collection was another point of discussion for a long time. A large part of the data was indeed obtained within the care system and was 'thus' primarily the responsibility and 'owned' by the paediatrician. Many parties built their own data collection to evaluate and publish. Around 2009 this situation was resolved by the construction of a central database 'NEORAH' (in full Neonatal Registration of Abnormal Dried Blood Spot Screening results), in which all clinical data can be entered by the paediatricians in shielded sections and for which agreements could be made about who has access to which data for reading and editing. Due to the fact that certain diseases occur very rarely, it is important that such a database exists for decades to collect sufficient data on diagnosis, treatment and follow-up. NEORAH went live on 1 November 2011. The success of this system obviously depends to a large extent on the willingness of those involved to carefully and fully enter the child's data.

Informing and Involvement of Professionals

A national screening programme can only function well if: everyone involved knows what diseases are in the programme and why; how important the information transfer is to parents for obtaining informed consent; how the heel prick blood samples should be obtained; why there is a certain time pressure for samples to be sent in time and analysed; and why the referral process to the paediatrician should be as short as possible. Although this sounds very logical today, but for years this was not so well organised.

Informing Parents/Guardians

Informing the parents should be a natural part of the antenatal care by midwives and further addressed by general practitioners and gynaecologists. However, due to lack of time and possible gaps in knowledge of the person taking the sample, for many years the heel prick information was given very little attention, while in the hospital the heel prick often just was 'done' without the parents knowing about it. Although many parents knew of the existence of the programme, they hardly understood what it was really about. As a matter of fact, this only changed at the large expansion of the programme in 2007, but it also had to do with social awareness in the field of health care that had been increasing over the years. The concept of informed choice was becoming increasingly important (Health Council 1989). It was clear that a short statement about the screening programme at the time of the heel prick was not enough. After some decades, the heel prick screening became routine so that information transfer received less attention and parents did not think much about it (Schipper 2008). Especially in the light of new enhancements, awareness was an issue that needed more consideration (Health Council 2005). Information about the nature of the disease, treatment options, but also the possible false positives, use of residual material from the heel prick and the fact that the heel prick is a voluntary choice might be more appropriate. It was noted that with regard to the choice, in practice there is some coercion or directivity because parents have a duty of care and are expected to act in the best interests of their child. If parents did not want to cooperate, the first step was to establish whether parents had sufficiently understood the information.

The question was also what the optimum moment in time was for providing more comprehensive information to the (future) parents. In the same Health Report (2005) it was advised to do this in the third trimester of pregnancy and repeat it briefly at the moment of sampling. However, the Royal Dutch Organisation of Midwives objected that at that stage all attention was focused on the upcoming birth. Alternatively, the time of routine ultrasonography, around the 20th week of pregnancy was proposed. Eventually the third trimester of pregnancy was chosen, in accordance with the advice of the Health Council. The Centre for Population Research developed a leaflet about the heel prick screening (and hearing screening) which is updated frequently (see Figure 2.5.).

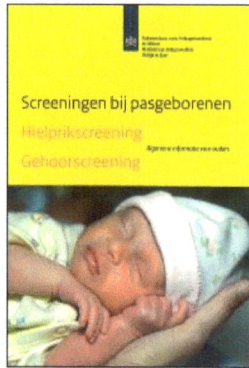

Figure 2.5. Information folder for expectant parents, 2013 edition.

Heel Prick Carried out by Different Professional Groups

At the start of the screening programme it was agreed that the staff of the nursing services would be responsible for the heel prick. In two provinces, *i.e.* Gelderland and South Holland, however, the agreement was that the midwives performed the heel prick as part of the follow-up of child delivery. The latter approach had two advantages: (1) Often the pregnant/young mother has a relationship of trust with the midwife, ensuring the information on the heel prick can be given in a calm environment and easier understood; (2) There was no need to wait for the notification of registration of the birth through the town hall office to the vaccination registries, before an employee of the nursing association could start to perform the heel prick. This shortened the process roughly one to two days. These two systems have always coexisted.

In 2006 it was decided that all newborns should undergo hearing screening. Until that time this was done at the clinic when the child was nine months old. For budgetary reasons, the Ministry of Health decided that the heel prick should be done whenever possible simultaneously with the hearing screening. The responsibility for both activities was assigned to the youth health care bodies by the Ministry. In Gelderland and South Holland the heel prick was then formally contracted to the midwives. In other parts of the country the screening is now usually carried out by so-called 'screen teams' composed of youth health staff who are specially trained in the heel prick (and hearing screening) and who must perform a minimum number per year to maintain their competence.

The Process of Referral

One of the delaying factors in the CH-screening process was the referral to the clinical paediatrician on the initiative of the provincial paediatrician (later called 'medical advisor of the vaccination registry'), via the general practitioner. Some general practitioners did not do this referral at all, but merely asked for additional diagnostics from the general practitioner's laboratory, others were slow in contacting the parents or making an appointment with the paediatrician. Because this was not the accepted practice in case of a referral for PKU, for which there had proven to be few false-positive results, the reason was probably partly due to the 'old' picture of there being a relatively large number of false-positive referrals, which existed in the early years of the CH-screening. Where necessary the Inspectorate gave admonishments, but the phenomenon has persisted. The National Steering Committee (LBC) considered therefore the solution to bypass the general practitioner in the referral process and to only inform him. That measure was inconsistent with the general health care policy for referral to the medical specialist and met with considerable resistance from the National Association of General Practitioners (LHV). That led to the incentive to invite the LHV to appoint a representative in the LBC.

Information to Practitioners of the Heel Prick

Despite all efforts over the years, one vital issue is still the timely puncture and the timely sending of the blood spot cards. In 1991, the RIVM obtained an American educational film on videotape. The RIVM also had an information brochure made by the firm Schleicher and Schuell (Figure 2.6.) translated into Dutch.

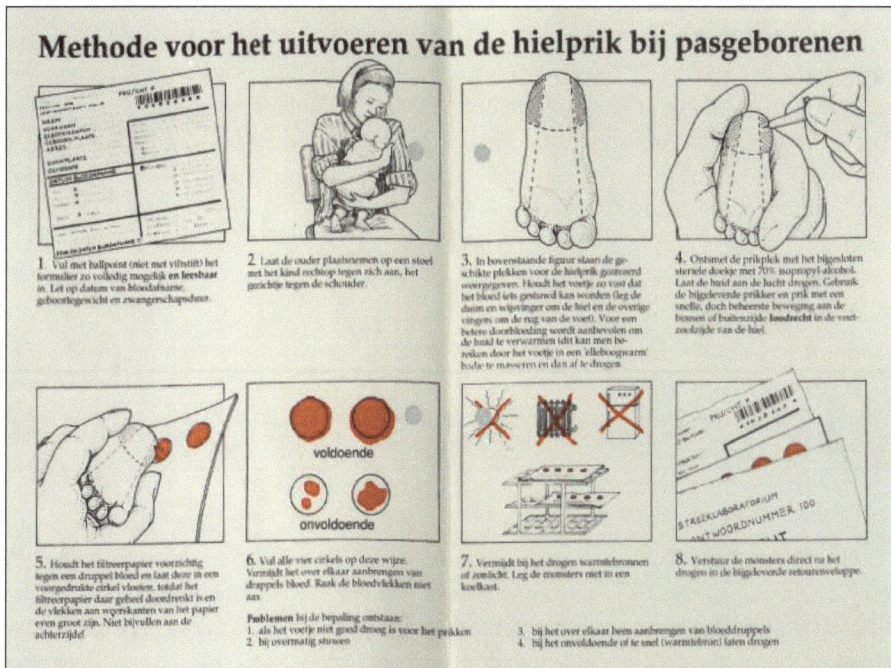

Figure 2.6. Information leaflet on performing the heel prick, front and middle sheet.

The videotape and brochure were used for instruction and briefings of employees of the vaccination registries and home care organisations to emphasize the importance of a good and timely executed heel prick. Yet there still was a need for a video that reflected the Dutch situation better, which in several respects is different from the American situation. Two such videos were produced in 2001, one for professionals and one for parents. Ten years later they were replaced with updated DVDs.

The ever-expanding programme also made the retraining of the practitioners necessary regarding the screened diseases. In the last ten years, the CvB, the Advisory Committees, the NVK and the Erfocentrum (a private organisation providing information about genetics of metabolic diseases) worked hard on the (electronic) availability of compact texts on the characteristics of each disease, while targeted information sessions for the various professional groups have been held (RIVM 2014b, Erfocentrum 2014). In the second half of 2013, the CvB moreover made an e-learning module available and the practitioners are also trained annually.

__News Item Published by the Centre for Population Screening, September 2013__
E-learning on heel prick screening
Every year about 180,000 newborns get a heel prick within the neonatal heel prick screening programme. Screeners who perform the heel prick have an important role in this screening programme.
From October 15, 2013, an e-learning module is available for screeners. In this e-learning module the whole process of the heel prick screening is addressed, such as informing the parents, birth registration, assignment for heel prick screening, obtaining parental consent, performance of the heel prick test, filling out the heel prick card, what to do with possible outcomes and the follow-up of abnormal screening results. After attending the e-learning module students have knowledge of the background and the correct implementation of the heel prick screening.
The e-learning is aimed at both screeners who perform the heel prick at home, and at health professionals who carry out the heel prick in the hospital, such as nurses and laboratory technicians.
Students need about 1.5 hours for the e-learning module. Students who pass the final test receive a certificate. The e-learning module is accredited by the professional associations of nurses and carers (V & VN) and midwives (KNOV).
More information is available at www.rivm.nl/hielprik/bijscholing.

Development Protocol

The above mentioned briefings illustrate how difficult it is to change ingrained habits. In the beginning of the PKU-screening it was thought that a minimum number of days of sufficient protein intake was essential for the proper functioning of the bacterial inhibition test. In practice it was shown that this assumption was not justified and that the heel prick could be carried out earlier. It was difficult to convince the screeners because "they had learned this in the past from their predecessors."

Changes in the screening programme or in the way of execution were incorporated into subsequent versions of the protocol for neonatal heel prick screening which, since 2006, is available online on the website of the RIVM (RIVM 2014c). During information meetings and from surveys it was evident that some practitioners unfortunately rarely consult this protocol (Van der Putten, 2005).

A persistent issue was the name 'PKU' for anything linked with neonatal screening. Thus, until the expansion in 2007, and even since then, many people still talk about 'PKU cards' when referring to the heel prick test cards; a '2nd PKU-test', even if a more common '2nd CH-test' was meant. This misuse resulted in additional administrative and analytical costs.

Another example is that blood is collected in hospitals not only for the neonatal screening programme but also for clinical diagnostic purposes often with cannulas with anticoagulants. Some anticoagulants are known to disturb the analysis in the screening laboratory. It was, and is, a burden to convince the staff in hospitals to not use these cannulas for the heel prick and to regard the heel prick test as a separate action.

Coping with Leftover Blood Samples

There was good agreement between the laboratories about the analytical methods used. However, there was no clear agreement about what to do with the remainder of the heel prick blood samples. Some laboratories discarded them shortly after completion of the analyses due to lack of storage space, some kept all cards for an indefinite period. In 1993 the Netherlands Society of Clinical Genetics requested the LBCs to keep all cards for a long time, e.g. five years, aiming for further scientific research. RIVM was regarded to be a suitable location. No further demands were formulated concerning the storage conditions, such as annealing temperature and humidity. After consultation with the RIVM, the LBCs agreed to the request.

Unclear Control

Actually, it was not clear who held the responsibility for the cards. This uncertainty was during the 1990s when more and more researchers wrote projects in which the prevalence of a (metabolic) disease, a genetic defect or the spread of an infectious disease could be examined. The LBCs were much in favour of most of the proposals, but did not know who should have the final decision. Most professionals favoured such role for the Health Inspectorate. Also the LBCs wanted to keep a finger in the pie, for example, to use blood spots for improvement of screening methods.

Besides anonymous prevalence survey studies there was also a demand for cards from individual children to perform diagnostics in view of a suspected congenital condition. The LBCs agreed to these studies provided that the researcher could show written permission from (one of) the parents.

> *Examples of anonymous prevalence survey: MTHFR folate; Smith Lemli Opitz syndrome; spinal muscle atrophy; the prevalence of congenital toxoplasmosis; the impact of dioxin on thyroid function; the spread of the swine flu virus. Examples of individual diagnostics: (1) When a child of a few years old had hearing impairment this could have been caused by a congenital cytomegalovirus infection; by going back to the blood of the heel prick card such connection could be confirmed. (2) When a second child in a family was found to have a disease (outside the screening program), and a previous child was deceased, sometimes such disease could still be diagnosed years later.*

New Civil Code (Medical Treatment Contracts Act)

In 1995, the new Civil Code part 7, was inaugurated. This included the Medical Treatment Contracts Act. Article 467 states that biological material can be used for other medical research if the donor has no objection.

> *Civil Code Article 467: 1. Human tissue and bodily secretions can be used for medical statistics or other medical research provided that the patient concerned has not objected to such research, and the research is carried out with the required care. 2. The term research is defined such that the human tissue and bodily secretions and the resulting data cannot be traced back to the patient concerned.*

That meant that from that moment on the parents had to give permission for storage. This change was not noticed within the LBCs. It meant that the long-term storage of blood spot cards for other research than the current screening programme was no longer in accordance with the law.

Enschede Firework Disaster

On May 13, 2000, a firework factory in Enschede exploded. As a consequence a number of people died. A journalist for the Trouw newspaper had heard of the stored blood spot cards and inquired at the RIVM if such cards could perhaps be used for identification of the victims. The text of the interview was pre-inspected and approved by the RIVM. See Figure 2.7.

Hielprik nuttig bij identificatie

Hans Marijnissen · 19/05/00, 00:00

Het Rampenidentificatieteam (RIT) dat in Enschede de identiteit vaststelt van gefragmenteerde lichaamsdelen van slachtoffers van de ramp, kan als dit kinderen betreft een beroep doen op een databank waarin de hielprikjes van 1,4 miljoen kinderen worden bewaard. Als het DNA-profiel uit een gevonden lichaamsfragment overeenkomt met dat uit een eerder afgenomen hielprik, staat de identiteit van het slachtoffer vast.

Op de lijst vermisten staat één kind van vier jaar. Sinds 1993 worden in Nederland alle kaartjes met bloed van een hielprik bewaard. Baby's krijgen op hun vierde tot zevende dag een hielprik, waarna een laboratorium onderzoekt of het kind lijdt aan een stofwisselingsziekte (PKU) of een afwijking aan de schildklier. Vanaf 1 juli worden pasgeborenen ook via het materiaal uit de hielprik gescreend op het erfelijke adrenogenitaal syndroom (AGS), dat kan leiden tot ernstig water- en zoutverlies en sterfte in de tweede levensweek.

De bloedmonsters die de huisarts, verloskundige of het ziekenhuis neemt, worden onder nummer doorgestuurd naar vijf laboratoria die onder controle staan van het Rijksinstituut voor volksgezondheid en milieu (RIVM) in Bilthoven. De resultaten worden doorgegeven aan de provinciale entadministraties, die de uitslag onder nummer koppelen aan het dossier van het kind

Zeven jaar geleden is besloten het kaartje met bloed niet langer weg te gooien, maar op te slaan bij het RIVM. Met 200000 geborenen per jaar is er inmiddels een bank ontstaan met gegevens van 1,4 miljoen Nederlanders. De bank kan medisch onderzoek dienen naar nieuwe ziekten, maar ook in individuele gevallen nut hebben: als een kind later een ziekte krijgt, kan worden bekeken of deze bij de geboorte al aanwezig was.

Het RIVM heeft geen zicht op de identiteit van de gescreende baby's. Het levert op verzoek van onderzoekers slechts een kaartje onder nummer. De honderdduizenden hielprikjes kunnen naarmate de bank groeit, in toenemende mate een rol gaan spelen bij moeilijke identificaties.

In de Verenigde Staten, waar in sommige staten al 30 jaar hielprikjes worden bewaard, is door zo'n bewaard monster zelfs een moord opgelost. In 1992 werden in Michigan de lichaamsdelen teruggevonden van de tienjarige Deanna Seifert, 63 dagen nadat zij was verdwenen. Het lichaam kon weliswaar worden geïdentificeerd, maar het lukte niet bloed uit het stoffelijke overschot te onttrekken, terwijl het kind ooit bloed had afgestaan. Toch was haar bloedgroep belangrijk, omdat de politie in de eerste dagen van de Deanna's verdwijning wel een verdachte had aangehouden met een druppel bloed op zijn schoen. Op basis van de hielprikgegevens kon de man uiteindelijk toch worden veroordeeld.

De hielprik mag in Nederland niet voor opsporingsdoeleinden worden gebruikt, omdat de bank voor louter medische doeleinden is ingesteld. Toch kan in uitzonderlijke gevallen een beroep op de bank worden gedaan, zoals bij vermissingen en rampen als in Enschede. Volgens justitie hebben ouders van vermiste kinderen de mogelijkheid toestemming te geven voor het opvragen van de hielprik, zodat deze kan worden vergeleken met op de rampplek aangetroffen sporen.

Figure 2.7. Text in the Trouw newspaper based on an interview with RIVM spokesman. Other media picked up the message (Figure 2.8.) and a turbulent period followed.

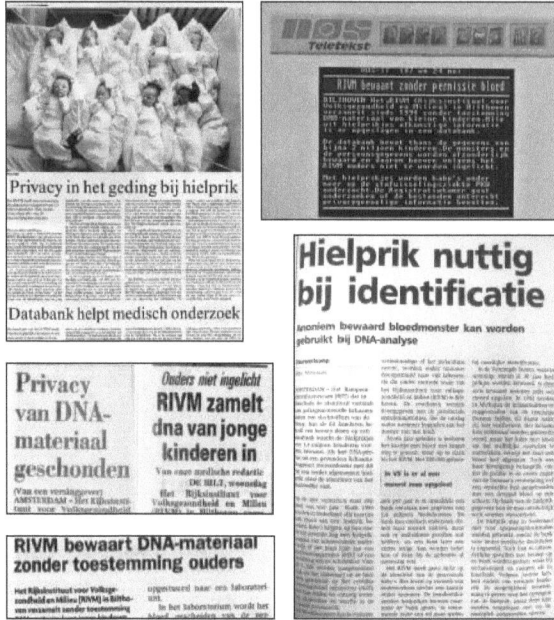

Figure 2.8. Examples of reports in the media following the fireworks disaster in Enschede on May 13, 2000.

Especially one heading of a televised message of the Netherlands national news agency (ANP) stating that "the RIVM collected DNA from babies" led to controversy among the general public. This heading was unnecessarily biased because there is a large difference between, on the one hand, the storage of the heel prick cards and, on the other hand, the very laborious and expensive isolation of DNA from each blood sample. Dozens of hate letters, phone calls and emails in which frequently comparisons were drawn with Nazi practices, followed. MPs asked questions of the Minister of Health. The Minister ordered an investigation by the (then) Registration Board (now Data Protection Authority), which came to the conclusion after several weeks that there was no evidence of an illegally structured data collection, but that the organisation of this storage was insufficient. The Registration Board further advised to put an advertisement describing the purpose of storage in a number of national newspapers (Figure 2.9.).

KENNISGEVING

OPSLAG HIELPRIKBLOED VANAF 1994 BIJ RIVM

Sinds 1974 wordt elk kind kort na de geboorte onderzocht op enkele aangeboren stofwisselingsziekten (PKU, CHT en AGS). Snelle opsporing daarvan is van groot belang om schade aan de lichamelijke en geestelijke ontwikkeling van het kind te voorkomen of te beperken. Per jaar worden tussen 80 en 100 kinderen opgespoord. Dit onderzoek vindt alleen plaats met toestemming van de ouders of verzorgers. Bij het kind worden met een hielprik enkele druppels bloed afgenomen. Dit bloedmonster wordt vervolgens in een laboratorium onderzocht. Het gehele screeningsprogramma wordt georganiseerd onder verantwoordelijkheid van de Provinciale entadministraties.

In 1993 besloten de LBC's (de medisch-wetenschappelijke commissies die het onderzoeksprogramma begeleiden) de bloedmonsters na het onderzoek op te slaan bij het Rijksinstituut voor Volksgezondheid en Milieu (RIVM) te Bilthoven. De bloedmonsters blijven daarmee beschikbaar voor de kwaliteitsbewaking van genoemde screeningsprogramma's en bovendien voor medisch-wetenschappelijk onderzoek, zoals anoniem onderzoek naar het voorkomen van andere stofwisselingsziekten. Hiervoor moet altijd eerst toestemming worden gevraagd aan deze begeleidingscommissies. Onderzoek dat herleidbaar is tot een individu (bijvoorbeeld indien een kinderarts in geval van ziekte van een kind wil nagaan of de ziekte reeds bij de geboorte aanwezig was) kan voorts alleen plaatsvinden na expliciete toestemming van de ouders of verzorgers.

De Registratiekamer heeft in augustus 2000 een rapport uitgebracht over de opslag van hielprikbloed bij het RIVM (www.registratiekamer.nl). De Registratiekamer beveelt onder meer aan de ouders of verzorgers te informeren over de sinds 1994 bestaande opslag van het hielprikbloed en hun de mogelijkheid te bieden alsnog bezwaar te maken tegen het bewaren van bloedmonsters van hun kind(eren) voor bovengenoemde doeleinden. Ook wordt aanbevolen om de informatiefolder die wordt uitgereikt voorafgaande aan de hielprik aan te passen. De aanbevelingen zullen worden overgenomen.

Ouders of verzorgers die meer informatie willen over de opslag van hielprikbloed bij het RIVM worden verwezen naar de internetpagina van het RIVM (www.rivm.nl). Verzoeken tot vernietiging van het hielprikmateriaal kunnen schriftelijk worden gedaan aan het RIVM t.a.v. dr. J.G. Loeber, Postbus 1, 3720 BA Bilthoven, onder vermelding van de naam en de geboortedatum van het kind. De vernietiging zal plaatsvinden onder toezicht van de Inspectie voor de Gezondheidszorg.

Namens de Landelijke Begeleidingscommissies,
prof. dr. R.C.A. Sengers, UMC Radboud, Nijmegen
Namens de Landelijke Vereniging van Entadministraties,
mr. P.A.A.M. de Hoogh, directeur, Bunnik
Namens het RIVM, dr. J.G. Loeber, Bilthoven

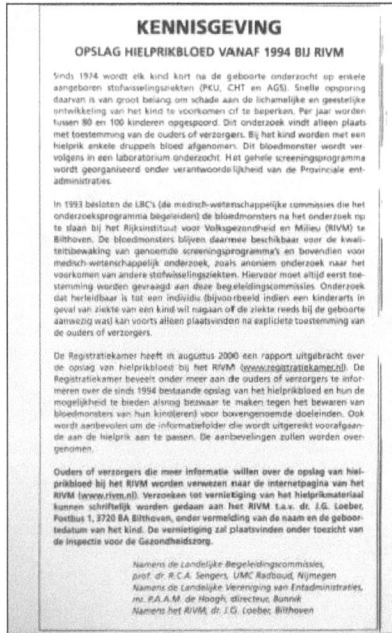

Figure 2.9. Communication in five national newspapers about the storage of blood samples in the RIVM.

Requests for Destruction

Parents who still wished to object could then make a request to destroy the heel prick card of their child. The number of parents that made such a request was relatively modest, about 550, but retrieval of these cards among the hundreds of thousands of others, plus the associated administration, was a heavy burden.

The LBCs proposed regulations on who the administrator of the cards would be, and who and under what conditions could obtain cards from the set, given the limited amount of residual blood. In addition, the LBCs demanded an endorsement of the research project by a medical ethics committee. The retention period of five years was (re-)defined. The text of the heel prick test sets was adjusted so that in future all parents could give their consent to the use of the heel prick card for anonymous research (Loeber, 2000). See Chapter 3 for a picture of the heel prick card.

After all the fuss had quietened down, the RIVM received the Big Brother Award 2002 awarded by the Foundation Bits of Freedom (Figure 2.10.).

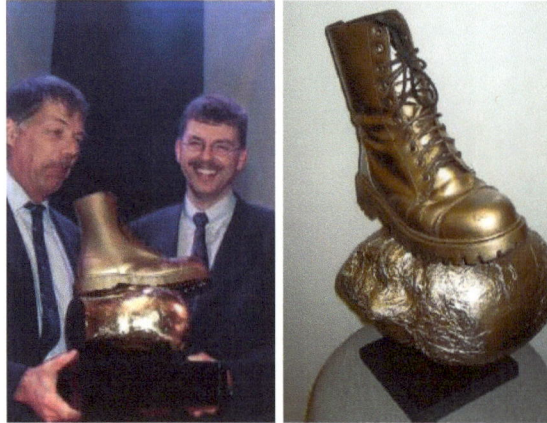

Figure 2.10. On the left Dr. J. G. Loeber (Head Reference Laboratory) and, on the right, Dr. D. Ruwaard (Director Division of Health) who, on behalf of the RIVM, received the Big Brother Award.

It should be noted that the discussion on residual human tissue: who the 'owner' is; who may decide to use it; how long it should be stored; and for which (scientific) goals; was not only going on in the Netherlands, but worldwide. Differences in legal and ethical attitudes in each country play a role (Bovenberg 2006). With the advent of genetic methods, it will be interesting to do long-term follow up studies of the changes in the genetic composition of the Dutch population. Researchers have proposed to periodically save a large selection of anonymous blood spot cards for decades under the right conditions for research and later release (ten Kate *et al.* 2005).

Automation

At the start of the screening when there were few or no computers, data administration was largely manual with forms and pencils. The daily laboratory screening results were recorded on the heel prick forms and sent by surface mail to the regional vaccination registries where they were copied into the register of all newborns: Awkward, cumbersome, time consuming and error prone (Rechsteiner 1979). From around 1980, there was some change. Every organisation, both vaccination registries and laboratories, developed a (semi-)automatic system, sometimes jointly with others, sometimes individually.

One of the first actions was in 1982, the RIV in 1982 made a computer terminal available with a printer to the Vaccination Registry Utrecht. Via a modem connection, contact could be made with the RIV main frame and lists of results (card numbers plus laboratory results) could be printed in the office of the vaccination registry. This reduced the paperwork in the screening laboratory and avoided the shipping process by surface mail. When it had been established to work well, from 1985 the RIVM attempted to get this introduced also in other parts of the country, supported by the simplification of the structure of the screening laboratories, first in 1986 and later again in 1995. After all, the screening process for every newborn in principle consists of a small number of the exact same steps: birth registration, signal to the screener, heel prick procedure, sending blood sample, laboratory analysis, sending the results to the vaccination registry, and if necessary, follow-up action.

The inventory in 1985, however, showed substantial differences between the procedures in municipalities, vaccination registries and laboratories (Loeber, 1986, 1987). Although all parties were convinced of the usefulness of the necessary harmonisation, the financial opportunities were limited, while it also remained unclear who had the authority to make decisions. Ultimately, the whole process of tuning and harmonisation lasted for about 10 years. In 2014, the RCP offices (former vaccination registries) have one common system (Praeventis) in which the child's data, obtained from the Central Population Administration, are linked to the results of neonatal screening and the national vaccination programme. The screening laboratories have a joint system (Neonat) in which the heel card numbers (sometimes supplemented with child data) are linked to the analytical results. The communication between the two systems also proceeds electronically with many safeguards for the preservation of privacy-sensitive information. Any change or extension of the screening programme implies that both systems should be adjusted.

Control by the LBCs

The National Steering Committees (LBCs) were faced with several practical issues. Usually, the discussions took place in a constructive atmosphere, but from time to time the interests and priorities of the various representatives of the professions and authorities concerned did not run parallel. Then the fact that the LBCs lacked decision-making powers became clear. Below is a short impression.

Extending the Birth Registration Period

In 1988 there was a proposal from some municipalities to extend the birth registration period from three to ten days. The LBC supported by the NVK wrote letters to the responsible Ministers of Justice and Health to emphasise the risk of losing effectiveness of the screening programme. Eventually the birth registration period remained unchanged at three days after birth.

Adjusting the Screening Model

From time to time the screening model was modified in an attempt to reduce the number of false-positive results, without increasing the number of false-negative results. Sometimes such decisions had profound implications for the agencies involved. So it was decided to change two things by early 1993. For premature infants, in the decision tree the age of sampling was no longer taken into account, and the concentrations of T4 and TSH were no longer expressed per punch of blood but per litre serum. Both led to modification of the software in the laboratories and vaccination registries. For these additional costs there was no central financial budget available. After some bickering about who should bear these costs, eventually the vaccination registries and the laboratories took care of it. It is an example of a good decision without considering all the consequences. This was the reason a working group was set up to check future changes with respect to legal and financial consequences.

Analytical Perils

Sometime after the introduction of the TBG determination, one of the five screening laboratories for unclear reasons yielded consistently higher results than the other laboratories. This meant a higher percentage of requests for second heel pricks and/or referrals. This naturally led to discussions within the LBC-CH and an urgent request to the RIVM (as reference laboratory) to find the cause. This was not found, but the discrepancy disappeared over time.

Furthermore, around 1997 a commercial bed-side kit for TSH in cord blood (Thyro Check) became available. This prompted some paediatricians to re-argue that the CH screening could now be carried out in this way with time savings as the main argument. Of course there were also arguments against this of which the cost increase by expanding the infrastructure was the most important, since the PKU and CAH screening had to continue using the heel prick blood sample. This is an example of how a screening programme for one disease cannot be separated from the total. After some discussion, the Thyro Check system was abandoned.

New Filter Paper

Since the beginning of the heel prick screening programmes in the 1960s, some countries used the filter paper "Schleicher and Schuell 903" (US, Australia, New Zealand), while in Europe and South America a different type was fashionable, namely "Schleicher and Schuell 2992". The main difference between the two grades was the blood absorption volume per volume of filter paper of about 20%. Within a programme this is not a problem but it hampered comparison of the results from different programmes, e.g. in external quality assessment schemes. In 1999, the company Schleicher and Schuell (later acquired by Whatman and now GE Healthcare) decided to gradually stop marketing type 2992 for neonatal screening. The transition to type 903 had to be prepared. After the manufacture and distribution of blood spot cards with the new filter by January 1, 2000, during many weeks the screening laboratories daily received a mixture of 'old' and 'new' cards which had to be well separated in order to correct the measurement results for the aforementioned 20% absorption difference.

Feedback on Negative Follow-Up Study

Any screening process unfortunately does not always run perfectly; sometimes there are sample mix ups or administrative errors occur. In 1999 it was decided that if the result of the confirmatory diagnostics of a referred child was negative, there always had to be a direct feedback to the referring screening laboratory to eliminate such errors. This procedure works well.

Dispatch of Heel Prick Cards by Mail

The Netherlands is a small, densely populated country with a good transportation infrastructure. Until the turn of the century the daily postal service was in the hands of a single company, PTT Post. During the development of the screening programme in the 1970s it was obvious to choose the mail service for the transport of the heel prick card with the blood samples. To save the screeners the hassle of loose postage stamps, a system of coded envelopes was chosen. Although every day the number of these coded envelopes had to be counted in the post office, this has not led to unacceptable delays in delivery. The heads of local post offices were informed of the medical urgency of the easily recognizable heel stick envelopes and therefore gave them priority.

However, PTT Post also went through changes. Between 2002 and 2011 the company was reorganized three times (in 2002 TPG Post; in 2005 TNT Post; in 2011 Postnl). Moreover, the daily amount of normal mail gradually reduced. Several times the organisational changes were found to have an impact on timely postal delivery. Each time it caused a search for the right person, at the right hierarchical level within the postal organisation, to gain understanding of the medical emergency and then to make that message also clear on a practical level.

Recently it was decided to modify the Postal Act such that from 2014 onwards, normal mail will not be delivered on Mondays anymore. For the screening programme a special arrangement is in place to secure the delivery of the heel prick envelopes at the screening laboratories on Mondays by using special medical weekend pillar boxes. In addition, the screening programme was faced several times with a strike of the postal service (1983, 1987, 2008, 2010, 2011) or a threat thereof, so that alternatives had be developed, e.g. a courier service like the one taking care of the distribution of daily blood and transfusion products throughout the country.

Children Born Abroad and Already Screened

Pregnant women who live in the border areas, sometimes go to hospitals in Belgium and Germany for the delivery. In 2000, the question was what to do with children who were born across the border and who had been screened there. Unfortunately, the screening programmes in each country differ in the selection of the diseases to be screened, particularly metabolic diseases, although there are also many similarities. The LBC considered that most metabolic diseases which had not been screened elsewhere already would have given rise to clinical symptoms at the time that the child returned to the Netherlands. The LBC therefore decided that the heel prick screening in the Netherlands should not be repeated unless the parents insisted.

Chapter 3: The Heel Prick Screening Programme in its Current Form

This chapter provides an overview of the screening programme as it exists in the year 2013. The entire screening process is described in the Protocol (RIVM2014b), and is diagrammatically represented in Figure 3.1.

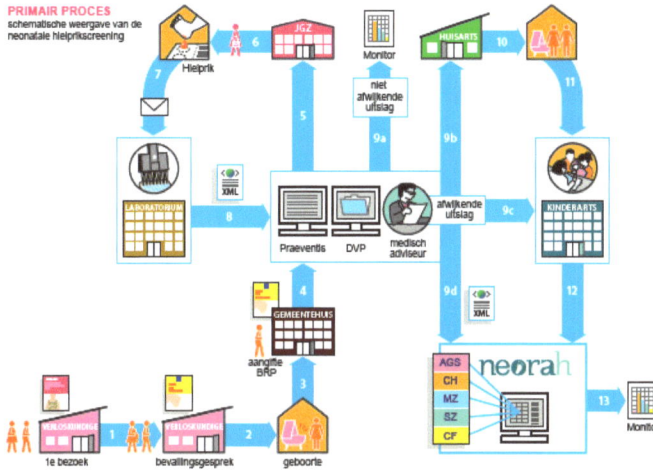

Figure 3.1. The heel prick screening process schematically.

The successive steps are roughly described in the following paragraphs.

Information during and Immediately after Birth

During pregnancy, the information to the pregnant woman is focused on all those aspects which should promote an undisturbed pregnancy. Things that take place after birth traditionally have not received much attention. However, with the advent of the internet and the growing need for information on many aspects of society, also the demand for sound information on the heel prick increased. There were concerns about the preservation of privacy and dispersal of genetic information of the newborn child. The currently selected solution is to provide general information at the beginning of pregnancy through the folder 'Pregnant!', and more detailed information when handing over the folder 'Screening programmes in newborns; heel stick screening and hearing screening' later in pregnancy. At the birth registration the father receives a folder containing the main features of the screening programme. In practice, right after birth the parents' attention is naturally on other things than the heel prick. Whoever performs the heel prick must make sure that the parents (or usually the mother) are (is) well informed to give consent, and therefore gives also a global summary, and may refer to other sources of information.

The Heel Prick in Daily Practice

The performer of the heel prick, nowadays often called 'screener', is given a so-called 'heel prick set'. This includes the following components:

1. A form on which the personal data of the newborn can be filled out; attached is a strip of filter paper on which a number of circles are printed; the form and filter strip have the same unique set number,
2. A punching device,
3. A Band-Aid or plaster,
4. A return envelope with the address of the regional screening laboratory,
5. An outer envelope with the same number as listed under 1 in which the items 1–4 are held together and can be kept by the parents as proof that the heel prick was performed.

The composition of the set in principle has not changed in 40 years, apart from a few details. Thus, in the 1990s the alcohol swab, with which the heel could be disinfected, disappeared because the risk of infection, at least in the home situation was considered negligible. The set number on the form and the filter strip is now also in barcode due to the automation of the process.

Filter Paper

The filter paper was replaced on the advice of the supplier in 2000 (Chapter 2). The size of the filter portion was adapted to the specifications of the analyser around 2005. The number of circles was increased in 2007 from four to six to stimulate the collection of more blood in connection with the expansion of the number of conditions to be screened for. The total surface of these six circles was about 20% greater than that of the previous four circles (Figure 3.2.).

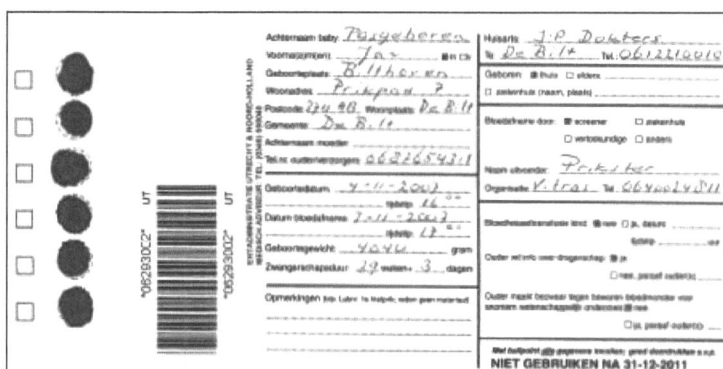

Figure 3.2. Image of a heel prick set 2007.

An instruction leaflet is available for the screener (Figure 3.3.).

HEELPRIKKAARTJE INVULLEN

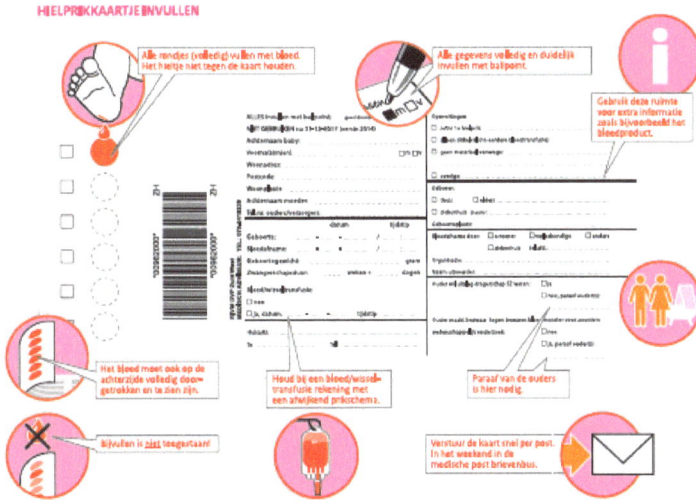

Figure 3.3. Instruction leaflet for performing the heel prick in 2014.

Puncture Device

Sampling of the heel blood was initially performed with a vaccinostyle, colloquially called the 'jenner' (Figure 3.4. a).

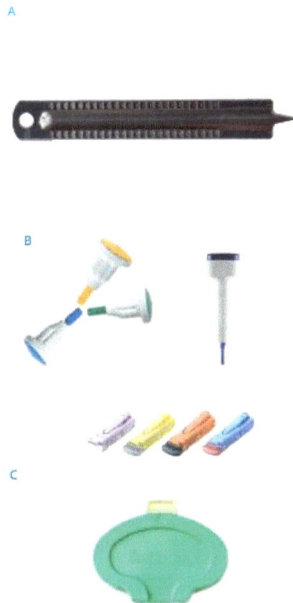

A

B

C

Figure 3.4. Various types of devices. (**a**) Traditional 'Jenner' from 1974–1990; (**b**) Various models from 1990–2006; (**c**) Current model 2007–present.

A jenner was a metal spike used in the past to infuse a small amount of vaccine in the skin, but which could also be used to obtain drops of blood. Provided that the heel was well warmed the jenner generally yielded enough blood. However, to save time warming the heel was often omitted and the jenner was blamed for the fact that insufficient blood was collected. Another (justified) objection was that the screener could injure himself on the sharp point of the jenner, which in the HIV era was no longer acceptable. The search for an alternative was not easy. One point of concern was the depth of the puncture because if it was in too deep there was a chance of osteomyelitis, an inflammation of the periosteum (Waelkens 1989). Several alternative devices (spring systems) were consecutively evaluated for their value, usually first within a pilot region, and then, when proven useful, applied nationwide (Figure 3.4. b). Optimally functioning devices did not puncture a hole but produced a very small incision, by which almost always enough blood was obtained. However, the cost has long been a major obstacle. Only after the expansion of the screening programme to include many conditions in 2007 and the increased need for blood volume, was that type put into operation (Figure 3.4. c).

> *Although the jenner has long since been abolished, for many years it was an indispensable part of the screening programme. In the 1990s, the RIVM has taken the initiative to honour people by awarding a Golden Jenner who for a long time had worked exceptionally for the success of the programme. Until 2014 this award has been given four times: to Rena Angulo-Laurent, Medical Advisor, Vaccination Registry, Utrecht (2005); Cor Verhaaff, Director, Vaccination Registry, Gelderland (2005); Gerard Loeber and Bert Elvers, RIVM Reference Laboratory (both 2012).*

In some foreign countries the suggestion has been made to obtain a blood sample via a puncture of the vein that runs on the back of the hand rather than a heel prick. This is supposed to be less painful for the baby, although hard evidence is lacking. A practical problem in the Netherlands is that puncturing veins ('venipuncture') can legally only be performed by certain medical professionals.

Heel Prick Set

The heel prick sets were ordered centrally once a year, produced and then delivered to the vaccination registries who took care of the distribution to the screeners and the hospitals. Due to the slow turnover it takes quite a long time for a change in the composition of the heel prick sets, or in the text on the form to be effected in practice. This was particularly difficult in the case of changing the filter paper (early 2000) after discussions about whether parents would consent to the medical scientific use of the residual blood samples (late 2000); and whether parents would like to have certain carrier information or not (2007).

These last two changes were not always well understood and led to discussion among screeners about what exactly the parents should be asked and whether they themselves or the parents should sign the form.

Technique of Blood Collection

The next step is the heel prick itself. In the early years the heel prick procedure belonged to a longer list of responsibilities of the nurse/health visitor. The technique was often learned from an older experienced colleague, with, unfortunately, erroneous habits such as the use of ointments that would promote blood flow. Some screeners had more problems getting enough blood and were then faced with a request from the screening laboratory to repeat the heel prick due to insufficient filling. From time to time, information sessions were organised for these professionals, with varying success.

Since 2007, the heel prick test is performed by a smaller number of screeners who need to do a minimum of a year to maintain the skill.

The Course of Events in and around the Screening Laboratory

Since the concentration of the screening to five regions on January 1, 1986, the screening laboratories receive daily between 100 and 200 blood spot cards, which are delivered by mail. The cards are sorted by province, checked for sufficient blood of sufficient quality and stamped with a serial number. The form with the demographic data is separated from the filter paper stub. The form will be read by the laboratory administration via the barcoded set number in the administrative software. The filter paper stub is processed in the laboratory, where the blood spots are punched and the punches processed in different analytical procedures. For many years punching was done manually with a special device. For medical-technical reasons this process was replaced by a (semi-)automatic device.

By soaking the punches in an aqueous liquid, the blood with the substances present are eluted. Subsequently, a part of the eluate is examined in an analytical procedure.

After approval, the measurement results of each analysis are coupled with the heel prick card numbers and reported electronically to the vaccination registries (DVP). The medical advisor then takes action for children with a screening result that could indicate the presence of a condition. This may lead to a second heel prick or a referral to the paediatrician.

Examples of Failures

Via the process described above, in 40 years some 7 million newborn children have been screened. Occasionally, an estimated 10–20 times per year, unfortunately something goes wrong.

- The child is not pricked because the family moved soon after birth and the child slips through all administrative cracks.
- The child will be pricked but the heel prick card is not sent, e.g. because the performer and the parents both think that the other party will take care of this.
- The child will be pricked, but the screener accidentally uses a heel prick set on which the demographic data of another child was already filled in, because on that day several children had to be pricked.
- The heel prick card arrives in time in the laboratory but there is too little blood of sufficient quality; there is a request for a repeat puncture but the screener forgets to do this or the parents refuse it.
- Two children are born on the same day and have exactly the same name.

- There is sufficient blood and all analyses are performed but the result is unfortunately incorrect so that a child is incorrectly referred or incorrectly not referred.
- The result is correct but does not reach the DVP-office.
- The results should lead to a referral but in that process something goes wrong.
- The results of two children are exchanged somewhere in the process and one child is incorrectly referred and the other is incorrectly not referred.

Three Real-Life Situations That Illustrate the Foregoing. (Names have been changed for privacy reasons).

1. A parent is going to make a book for her daughter who is already 14 months old. There is a photo taken during the heel prick procedure in the hospital. In the picture you can see the girl lying in her bed. There is a visible hand holding the heel prick test kit. Because it is so nice to be able to read the data of the child in the picture, the mother zooms in on the clear data entered and finds that these belong to another baby, even a boy! Panic everywhere, mother contacts the hospital and the medical advisor DVP. Checking the database yields that a total of four children had a heel prick done on that day in the hospital. Fortunately, all the results of the four children prove to be normal. It is important that the parent, if possible, checks the demographic data entered on the heel prick form.

2. There is an abnormal result in a child 'Marilyn Monroe' located in the Radboud Hospital in Nijmegen, born on October 1, which according to data on the heel prick card is a resident of Arnhem. The screening laboratory reports its results to DVP-East in Deventer. The employees look for a Marilyn Monroe, born on October 1. Such an unusual name must still be easily retrievable. Yes, this child turns out to live in Boxmeer, on the other side of Nijmegen, a region that is overseen by DVP-South. On the heel prick cards frequently the address where the infant (temporarily) stays is noted instead of its formal residential addresses. The young mother will stay (with child) for example a while with her parents. Given that this is such an 'exclusive' name, one assumes that it is one and the same child. A request for referral is put in motion by region DVP-South. Gradually it becomes clear that two children with this exclusive name were born on the same day, one of which (the child with the abnormal result) had not yet been registered in the software database Praeventis. DVP-employees must not only act on the (exclusive) name of the child but also check the other demographic information and always take into account that it could be another child.

3. The screening programme includes sickle cell disease (SCD), the method also identifies carriers. This condition is really only prevalent in children of parents with African, Mediterranean or Asian background. On a certain day, the screening laboratory reports results for two SCD carriers for two children named: Pietje Jansen and Elsje de Boer. The administrative assistant with years of experience in the screening programme has a hunch. Usually children who are SCD carriers have names with a non-indigenous sound. She brings this to the attention of the medical advisor who contacts the screening laboratory to discuss this. Could there be a mix-up in the laboratory? And yes, that turns out to be so. The real carriers indeed have a non-native name.

In short, several situations where a basically simple process can go wrong. For each situation, a system of check and double check has been invented but that system should be regularly tested for its robustness. Using these checks, the number of children without a proper screening result is very limited.

Check Measures

The analytical quality is monitored daily in the laboratory (see below).

The DVP staff perform a completeness check: for every newborn all screening results must be in the system by 18 days after birth. In the absence thereof the cause will be investigated and, if possible, a heel prick still carried out.

For most conditions, it is essential that the results are obtained rapidly and, if abnormal, that the referral happens quickly. In the early days of the PKU screening, then using the bacterial inhibition assay, the reading of the growth zones sometimes led to mistakes. This prompted the reference laboratory in the RIVM to periodically send dummy samples around with elevated phenylalanine concentrations; thus leading to an abnormal result being sent to the laboratories. The intention was to keep the laboratory technicians on their toes. These dummy samples were indistinguishable from the rest of the daily samples. The name of the baby and the rest of the data were fictitious. The DVP offices were warned in advance that a dummy would be circulated so that when notified of the abnormal result, no further steps would have to be taken by the laboratory. The RIVM registered if all screening laboratories had identified these samples and how long it had taken to notify the DVP-offices.

This system with dummy samples has operated for many years. It went wrong once when, with it being on a weekend, the then South Holland Vaccination Registry had transferred its 'service' to the then Vaccination Registry Rotterdam, but had failed to warn them that the result of a dummy sample was underway. When the abnormal result was reported by the laboratory, the employees of the Vaccination Registry Rotterdam searched in vain for the fictitious child at the fictitious address and even the police were called in to help in the search.

Clerical errors in the registration of the results unfortunately happened a few times. For the incorrectly referred child, the abnormal screening result could then not be confirmed (In fact, all blood values were then completely normal, which is different from a more common false-positive screening result). This led to a change in the protocol that, in such a case, the attending paediatrician must contact the referring screening laboratory immediately to ascertain what the cause of the discrepancy might be. In all cases of mistaken identity, the incorrectly non-referred children were seen by the paediatrician after all.

Due to ongoing automation and especially due to positive sample identification through barcodes, the most 'simple' errors virtually ceased or they are much faster detected and corrected than in the past.

Laboratory Analytical Methodology

Most readers will not, or only partially be familiar with, the ins and outs of the analytical methods used in the heel prick screening. To lift a corner of the veil and for a better understanding of paths some policy decisions follow, the essentials are highlighted below.

Bacterial Inhibition Assay

This method makes use of the growth of the bacterium Bacillus Subtilis on an agar plate. The growth is inhibited by adding a certain concentration of the substance beta-2-thienylalanine. In the presence of an increased concentration of the phenylalanine, this inhibition is overcome and the bacterium will still grow. For the analysis, a punch of the filter paper with blood is placed on the agar. Blood components, including phenylalanine, are extracted into the agar. After an overnight incubation, one sees a zone of growth around the punch, the diameter of which is proportional to the concentration of phenylalanine (Figure 3.5.). By putting a number of punches with increasing known amounts of phenylalanine on each agar plate, and measuring the diameters of the growth zones, a calibration curve can be obtained with which the concentration of phenylalanine in the samples from newborns can be calculated.

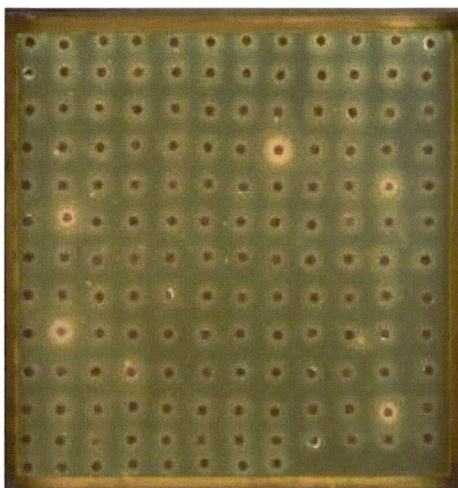

Figure 3.5. Agar plate with blood punches. Around the punches with high phenylalanine concentration a growth area is visible.

The advantage of this method is the low cost; there are no complicated and expensive reagents or equipment required. The disadvantage is its laborious nature. In order to avoid that, besides the phenylalanine, also blood proteins from the punch extract in the agar and disrupt the reading, all the strips of filter paper are first heated in an autoclave or a microwave oven.

There is also a chance of errors in the reading of the growth zones, the influence of components in the blood sample which inhibit the growth of bacteria, such as residual antibiotics, and the fact that automation is virtually impossible. Nevertheless, the Netherlands has used this method from 1974 to 1995. Many developing countries still use the method because of its low cost. Figure 3.6. shows the successive steps of this method.

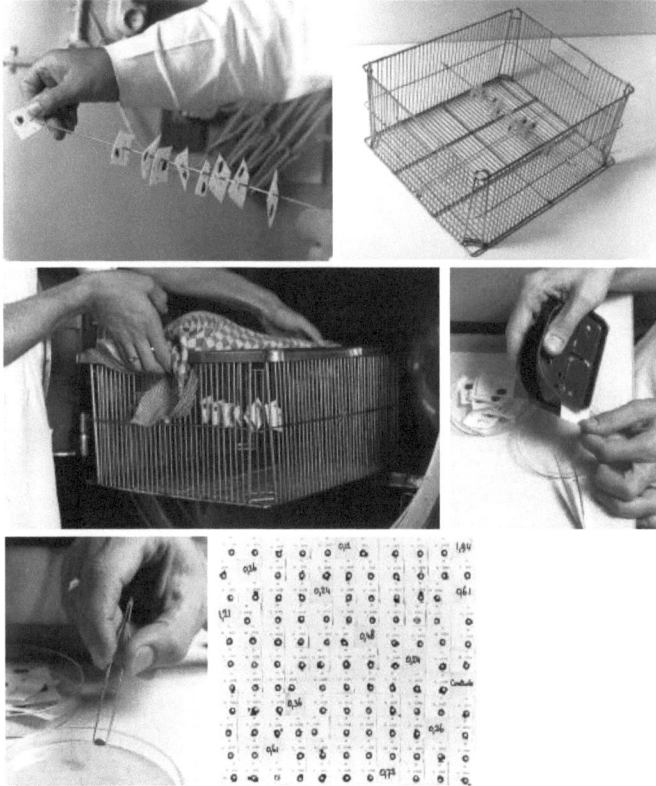

Figure 3.6. Execution of a bacterial inhibition assay. The filter paper stubs are strung on a wire and hung in a wire basket. The wire basket is heated in an autoclave. With a perforator, a punch is taken from a blood spot, and the punch is put on the agar plate with the aid of a pair of tweezers. After an overnight incubation, growth zones are visible. The site of the punches corresponds to the filter paper stubs that were stuck on a sheet of paper, so that it is clear which punch belongs to which infant.

Enzymatically-Colourimetric/Fluorometric Methods

In the body, phenylalanine normally is converted to tyrosine by the enzyme phenylalanine hydroxylase. This reaction can also be carried out in the laboratory. The reaction mixture consists of an eluate from the blood punches, containing the phenylalanine to be measured, the enzyme phenylalanine hydroxylase, and a number of additives. After incubation, during which the enzyme is doing its job, a colour is formed (Figure 3.7.) or a product which fluoresces. The intensity of the colour or fluorescence can be measured in a measuring device developed for this purpose and compared to that of a series of blood samples with known levels of phenylalanine.

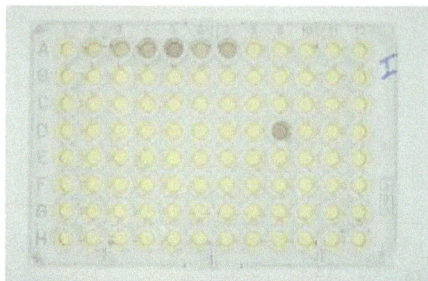

Figure 3.7. Microtiter plate after completion of the assay. A yellow colour indicates a low-, a brown colour a high-phenylalanine concentration in the original blood sample.

The advantages and disadvantages are complementary to those of the bacterial inhibition test, *i.e.,* more expensive due to the reagents and the required device, but faster, less error-prone and automatable.

The principle of enzymatic colorimetry is also the basis of the assays for biotinidase deficiency and galactosemia.

Immunochemical Methods

In the Netherlands, for congenital hypothyroidism, the concentrations of thyroxine (T4), thyrotropin (TSH) and thyroxine-binding globulin (TBG) are measured. In immunochemistry, use is made of an interaction between an antigen and an antibody raised against that antigen. Over the years, several variant embodiments have been developed, but the oldest one is the radio immunochemical method, in which the antigen (e.g. TSH) is mixed with radioactively-labelled TSH and antibodies against TSH. Both forms of the antigen bind to the antibody. Therefore, the reaction mixture contains the eluate from the blood punch (containing TSH), an amount of radioactive TSH and an undersized anti-TSH.

Over time, the antibody-bound TSH is separated from the non-bound TSH. In the bound fractions, the radioactivity is measured in a gamma counter. The more TSH there is in a sample, the less radioactive TSH has a chance to be bound to the anti-TSH. This is again made visible with a set of blood samples having known amounts of TSH. There is a decreasing calibration curve, from which the TSH concentration can be calculated in the heel prick blood samples. Over time the radioactivity has been replaced by an enzyme, in which the end point of the method shifted from the amount of radioactivity to the colour intensity of an unreacted substance by the enzyme. Still later, a variant was marketed in which the enzyme was replaced by a fluorescent marker. By making use of different markers more than one component in a blood sample, for example T4 and TSH, can be measured at the same time. Such simultaneous determination saves time, and uses less of the small amount of the blood samples available.

Immunochemical methods have also been applied to the screening for congenital adrenal hyperplasia (via the measurement of the concentration of 17α-hydroxyprogesterone), and for cystic fibrosis (concentration of immunoreactive trypsinogen and pancreatitis-associated protein).

High Performance Liquid Chromatography (HPLC)

Chromatography is a technique in which molecules are separated from each other on the basis of their size and/or of their electric charge. Over time various methods have been developed, such as paper chromatography and thin layer chromatography. In HPLC, a mixture, in this case the eluate of a punch, is forced through a column under high pressure. The molecules adhere to the column material for a shorter or longer period of time and are thus separated from each other. HPLC is used in the screening for sickle cell disease. Different molecular forms of haemoglobin are separated from each other. We are particularly interested in the question of whether, in addition to the ordinary forms of haemoglobin, such as the so-called foetal haemoglobin and the adult haemoglobin, also haemoglobin S is present in the blood sample, because it is characteristic of sickle cell disease. In the separation step also other forms of haemoglobin may be found. The ratio of the concentrations of all of these forms indicate whether or not there is a need for further diagnostic examination by the paediatrician.

Tandem Mass Spectrometry

This is currently by far the most advanced technology. The name indicates that the device has two mass spectrometers (ms/ms) in sequence ('in tandem') stand. The eluate from the punch is placed on the apparatus. The molecules are separated into the first mass spectrometer by size and charge, and then broken into pieces in the 'collision chamber'. The fragments are finally separated from each other in the second mass spectrometer. This technique allows us to simultaneously measure the concentrations of dozens of substances which are indicative of certain diseases. At higher concentrations, there is reason to refer the child to the paediatrician for further diagnosis. In the current programme it involves metabolic diseases of fatty acids, organic acids and amino acids. In the past, the ms/ms technique has been developed primarily for the detection of medium-chain fatty acid dehydrogenase deficiency (MCADD). However, also PKU can be detected with this and that made the application of the aforementioned methods for PKU superfluous.

Whole Genome Sequencing (WGS)

This technique means that the DNA sequence of the newborn is mapped out completely. This technique is not used yet, but is considered by some experts as the ultimate approach because all genetic defects can be detected at once. With rapidly expanding technological capabilities, the cost of the analysis will fall rapidly, though it will still be much higher than that of the currently used screening techniques.

Introduction of this WGS technique in the neonatal screening programme, however, is problematic for several reasons. Conditions may be detected that manifest themselves later in life or are untreatable, which is not in accordance with the current scope of the heel prick screening where the emphasis is on health benefits for the child in accordance with the criteria of Wilson and Jungner. Other problems would be to identify the multitude of genetic data, since not from all the genetic variants are the biochemical effects precisely known. Therefore, a lot of different biochemical analyses would have to be carried out to confirm or deny the presence of the condition.

Finally, a solution has to be found to the problem of how additional genetic information that is obtained at the same time can be kept confidential (Health 2010b).

Quality Control

The diversity of technology requires tight daily quality control. For this, the laboratories use statistical methods that are common in clinical chemical laboratories. Analytical quality is monitored through a system of internal quality controls in which, for each measurement series, a number of samples with known concentrations are processed. In addition, each laboratory participates in a system of external quality assurance in which an independent organisation circulates samples of which the concentration is not known in advance. The laboratory reports the results and will be told later whether they were correct within certain limits. In case of erroneous results for a certain method, a quick consultation between colleagues from other screening laboratory can be implemented to see if similar abnormalities have occurred there as well. If necessary, the supplier of the equipment and/or reagents can be consulted.

In addition to the analytical quality, also the turnaround time is monitored. Further, the laboratories report their results quarterly to the reference laboratory followed by an open discussion about the combined results. All parameters are summarized in periodic reports, which has in the past been done quarterly (Schopman *et al.*1981–1990), and at present annually (Loeber *et al*. 1991–2006; Elvers *et al*. 2006–2012).

Procedure in the DVP Offices

Registration of Births

Every newborn in the Netherlands is registered at the Department of Population of the local municipality and subsequently included in the national Registration of Persons. In the past, the local municipalities reported daily all births to the then provincial vaccination registry by surface mail and later by fax. In Amsterdam, often an extra day was needed because the messages from the sub-municipalities were first collected at a central point. Another source of delay were the so-called 'incidental births'. These were children who were born in one province but lived in a different province. The provincial vaccination registry then had to forward the message to the appropriate provincial vaccination registry.

A big step forward was the digitalisation of the national birth registry and the fact that the provincial vaccination registries were allowed online access to it in order to pick up the birth reports for their area. In the 1990s the vaccination registries decided to replace their separate computer systems by a common software package called 'Praeventis'. Each newborn's personal data are included in Praeventis. Later, not only the data on performed vaccinations but also the results of the heel prick screening were added in this system.

Notification for Heel Prick to Youth Health Care

After receiving the announcement of the birth at the vaccination registry, a notification is given to the office of Youth Health Care in the particular municipality. An employee visits the family, explains the screening programme and, after receiving permission, performs the heel prick using a specially developed set (see above). For children who are still in the hospital at the time of the heel prick, this is performed by hospital staff.

Each heel prick set has a unique number. The heel prick card is sent to the screening laboratory, which forwards a copy of the form with the personal data and heel prick card number to the DVP-office; in the past by surface mail or by fax, today mostly electronically. The DVP-office now has the link between the infant's name and the set number and can add this number to the data of the child in Praeventis. If one or two days later, the screening results with the set number are received from the laboratory, the results may also be added in Praeventis.

In over 98% of the children, the screening process is then completed. In about 1.5%, the first screening results are not unequivocally abnormal or normal, but so-called 'dubious'. Then a second heel prick test must be performed by the YHC or hospital. In 0.4%, one or more screening results are abnormal and the infant is referred to the paediatrician for confirmatory diagnostics and possible treatment.

Role of the Medical Advisor

While the DVP-employees have an important task to complete the registration of all data on time, the medical advisor has the medical responsibility for assessing the screening results and deciding on a second heel prick or a referral. In case of a referral, the medical advisor tries to contact the family doctor and asks him to inform the parents about the referral. The medical advisor usually already has contacted the paediatrician, except in the case of CH, because then the parents and the family doctor choose the paediatrician. The paediatrician reports the results of the diagnostics to DVP and TNO (see above) in view of the annual evaluation of the programme.

This is the situation on paper, but in practice it is more complicated. Formally, the family doctor is the gateway to the paediatrician. However, some young families, especially in the big cities, do not (yet) have a family doctor. Even today many doctors work part time so that the identification of the general practitioner or his substitute takes time. 'Time' is the biggest bottleneck because referrals based on an abnormal screening result are always urgent and preferably should take place on the same day. In practice, a family doctor is rarely confronted with an abnormal screening result. It is not surprising that they are not aware of all the details of all screened diseases. Some believe that the help of a paediatrician is not necessary, and that they themselves may be in a position to take care of the follow-up diagnostics. For the medical advisor it is sometimes quite a challenge to lead this process properly. If there is no family doctor available, the medical advisor will contact the parents. They will then have to be convinced of the need to take the seemingly healthy child quickly to a paediatrician. Especially young fathers do not want to accept that message from a medical adviser. He therefore has a duty to check after a few days or a week, if the child has actually been seen by a paediatrician.

Diagnosis after Referral

Usually, the medical adviser first contacts the academic paediatric clinic, respectively CF centre, in the region of residence of the child. For congenital hypothyroidism (CH) the procedure until now is that the child is referred to a paediatrician chosen by the parents (see above). If the relevant clinic/paediatrician is unavailable, then the medical advisor will look for an alternative. Depending on the screening results as to what the condition is, the appointment with the paediatrician is on the same day or the next day.

The child is physically examined and blood and urine samples are taken. If the diagnostics confirm the screening result, the child will undergo treatment, either in the clinic or elsewhere.

Sometimes the diagnostics show that the screening results were false positive. Although the parents in such a case initially may be irritated or angry, practice shows that this period lasts only briefly, especially if the paediatrician can explain it carefully. There are no indications of a permanent sense of anxiety or a different type of parent–child bonding, contrary to what was described previously (Tijmstra 1984). Usually the contact with the paediatrician ends here.

The results of the diagnostics are processed in databases developed for this purpose (NEORAH resp. DDRMD (Dutch Diagnosis Registration Metabolic Diseases)). This information may help to determine whether the screening system should be changed by adjusting the alert limits of the analysis result, or by switching to the measurement of more or alternative components in the blood samples. Children with a determined disease remain under the care of a paediatrician for a long time, sometimes decades, and in some situations subsequently an internist. It would be good to also record the results of the long-term follow-up in databases to get an idea how screening and timely diagnostics and treatment really contributed to good health. Due to the small number of patients per disease per year, it can take years before comparative medical research can draw clear conclusions. It is well conceivable that some apparent conditions, over time, can be considered to be a natural variation, and could be in fact taken off the screening panel. An example is histidinemia which in a number of countries has been screened for many years, though not in the Netherlands. Also, doctors, out of precaution, will want to treat or monitor diagnosed persons permanently which will give them the stamp 'patient' thus having an impact on their quality of life. Sometimes, after the addition of a condition to the screening panel, the prevalence appears to be much higher than previously thought, possibly due to over diagnosis or mild cases. Perhaps mild cases should not be labelled as "a patient".

In the current situation, such long-term results are not easily retrievable and interpretable. In recent years the Ministry of Health has made available funding for developing NEORAH Phase 2: Long Term Follow Up on Heel Prick Screening. In 2013, a first start was made in inputting data for CAH and sickle cell disease.

Results of 40 Years of Screening

The table below shows the main results of (almost) 40 years screening (the figures for 2013 were not yet known at the time of writing). The numbers have been derived from the annual reports of TNO (Verkerk et al., 1991–2012) and from data published elsewhere (Verkerk et al. 1993, Verkerk 1995, Lanting et al. 2005). In some situations, the precise diagnosis at the time of reporting was not yet known, therefore the reported numbers contain a degree of uncertainty. However, this table is primarily intended to indicate the order of magnitude for each of the screened (group of) clinical pictures. The calculated prevalences here, i.e. the ratio between the number of confirmed diagnoses and the number of screened children, are generally consistent with the values expected based on foreign data.

Table 3.1. Results of 40 years of screening (column headings: period, births, screened, referred, confirmed, prevalence).

	Periode	Geboorten	Gescreend	Verwezen	Bevestigd	Prevalentie
PKU	1974-2012	7.161.669	7.124.956	860	493	1:14.452
CH-T					1968	1:3063
	1981-2012	6.055.454	6.028.360	19.921		
CH-C					256	1:23.548
AGS	2002-2012	2.072.976	2.064.258	440	118	1:17.346
MZ				1256	315	1:3480
SCZ					215	1:5098
α-Thal	2007-2012	1.100.655	1.096.269	484	195	1:5621
β-Thal					24	1:45.677
CF	2011-2012	252.974	252.188	66	49	1:5146

The table shows that the percentage of children screened is greater than 99.5%. Reasons for not participating in the screening programme are: the child dies before screening takes place, refusal of parents, or moving abroad. In nearly 40 years, more than 23,000 children have been referred for further diagnosis. Over 3600 children have been treated.

From time to time an affected child is missed by the screening programme if the concentration of the blood parameter falls inside the 'normal' area. This is known as a false negative result. Sometimes this becomes apparent only years later on the basis of clinical symptoms or family history research, if a brother or sister born later is found to have the disease. The number of children with a false-negative screening result was estimated in previous long-term overviews at 2% for PKU (Verkerk, 1995) and 1% for CH (Verkerk *et al.* 1993); it is expected that these percentages have declined slightly in recent years due to tightening of the cut off limits. For other diseases, there are not (yet) enough statistically reliable data.

The Opinions of Parents

It is striking that between the start of the screening programme in 1974 and the 'big' expansion in 2007, parent and patient organisations have not been represented in the national consultative bodies, such as the aforementioned National Steering Committees. This may be due to the changing role of patients in general: the patient has become more articulate and will not take anything for granted any more.

It makes a difference whether we talk about parents in general, or parents with a child whose health is threatened in any way. Fortunately, the latter group is much smaller. By organising themselves into associations, these parents are better able to put their views forward. So we now know of, amongst others, the Association Adults, Children and Metabolic Diseases, the Dutch Phenylketonuria Association, the Foundation 'Schild' (congenital hypothyroidism), the Dutch Association for Addison's and Cushing's patients, Oscar Netherlands (sickle cell disease), the Dutch Cystic Fibrosis Foundation and the umbrella organisation Genetic Alliance (VSOP). Some of these associations are represented with temporary or permanent committees that advise on the establishment, improvement and possible expansion of the neonatal screening programme.

Parents with an affected child have experience and expertise and they can indicate very well where the health care system, including the neonatal screening programme, is inadequate and how it can be improved. This applies to individual diagnosis, how a possible referral to a paediatrician should be communicated and what information is appropriate at each stage of the process. Participation of patients' organisations in the screening programme committees since 2006 (see Chapter 2) has therefore been a welcome addition. Based on their own experiences with patients, parents often have ideas about which diseases should or should not be included in the screening programme, and sometimes they interfere publicly in discussions about expanding the programme (VSOP 1999; Reerink 2007; van den Berg, 2007).

Policymakers need to explore new possibilities, but must also be able to argue that sometimes there is a limit to the technical and financial capacity, and to explain moral principles underlying the choices made. This is a continuous process because the technical possibilities, both in detecting diseases and in the diagnosis and treatment, constantly shift and because therefore the principles of screening must always be reaffirmed or perhaps adjusted. New developments often get a lot of attention in the media awakening expectations with parents and the general public that cannot always be realized in large-scale application in a prevention programme. Sometimes the treatment is still uncertain, or the test is too unreliable, causing the disadvantages at the population level to outweigh any advantages. This then leads to frustration among the parents of the children involved.

It is important that screening programmes, with all the possibilities and impossibilities, receive regular attention in the media and in teachings at school, so that the basic knowledge is rooted in society without false expectations. This would also boost further discussions and opinion making on neonatal screening. In addition, social science and ethics research contributes to mapping opinions of parents and reflection on new developments so that they are clear to policy makers (Detmar *et al.* 2008; Tijmstra *et al.* 2008; Plass *et al.* 2010; Weinreich *et al.* 2012; van den Burg and Verweij 2012). This would all help in the decisions regarding important issues facing the programme in the coming years.

New techniques will increase the possibilities to find conditions that are difficult or impossible to treat, or that manifest themselves later in life. In the case of untreatable disorders, some parents would like to receive more information, while others would not want to miss the relatively carefree time with their child. Also, not everyone will want to use the results of the heel prick screening for reproductive choices in a subsequent pregnancy. The danger is that by such further (new) opportunities, the programme will deviate from its core mission, namely a public facility to prevent serious diseases in newborns. In addition, for some parents such expansions would be a reason for not being willing to participate in the programme, which would be a risk for public health.

Chapter 4: Newborn Blood Spot Screening in Other Countries

Shortly after the publication of Guthrie on his method to detect PKU in blood samples, various countries set their own screening programme on track. The first were New Zealand, the United Kingdom, Sweden and Switzerland in 1965. Via publicity through scientific journals and conferences more countries became interested. It is not surprising that especially the richer and more developed countries started the process quickly while in other countries it took more time, even decades, before they had the opportunity to start. Figure 4.1 shows the onset for other European countries.

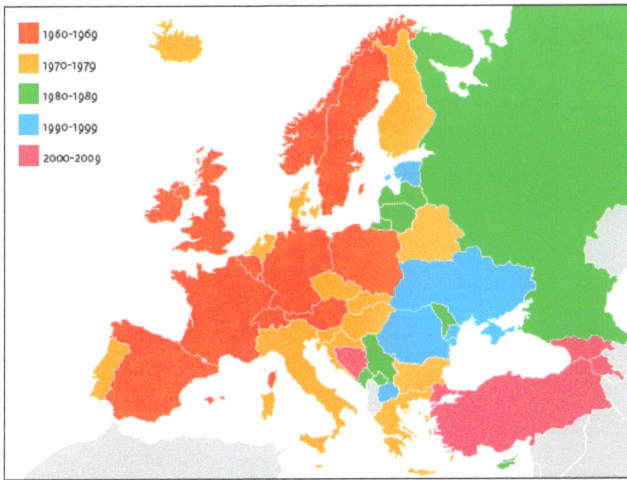

Figure 4.1. Decade in which the country has launched a (more or less) regular screening programme.

At the time of writing in 2013, however, there are still many parts of the world where neonatal screening is still not on the policy makers' agenda, usually because of lack of money and other health care priorities. It is estimated that only about 30% of all newborn babies in the world are screened.

In countries that screen, there are major differences visible in the choice of which conditions to screen for. Almost everywhere PKU and CH have been given priority. That obviously has to do with the enormous burden of disease that can be prevented, the rate of occurrence in the population and the relatively simple detection methods and treatment of affected children, although in some countries there are debates as to who should bear the costs of the PKU diet. The choice of further conditions after these first two often leads to heated discussions between the professionals involved in each country, usually paediatricians and geneticists. However, also the establishment and financing of health care in a country play an important role in further expansion.

Situation in the United States

In the US, the states in principle are independent in their policies, while the federal government can do no more than give recommendations. However, public opinion also plays a large role. Eventually the citizens of any particular state sees himself as an American and looks with great interest to what happens in states other than his own. In the 1990s the newspapers were full of indignant articles that showed significant differences in the selection of the screened conditions. 'How is it that a child born on one side of a state border is screened on many more or less conditions than a child born on the other side?' In 2003, the American College for Medical Genetics (ACMG) was commissioned by the federal government to make an inventory of what each state was doing, as well as a survey of domestic and foreign colleagues for their opinion about priorities for expansion. In 2006, the report was published. A list of 29 conditions was recommended as first priority ('recommended uniform screening panel (RUSP)', Watson *et al.* 2006). All States were urged to comply which was effected around 2010. Meanwhile the RUSP had been supplemented with three new diseases, *i.e.* Severe Combined Immunodeficiency (SCID), Critical Congenital Heart Disease and Pompe's disease. It is expected that in a few years all states will have implemented screening for these three as well.

Situation in Europe

In Europe, the picture is totally different. In general, one can say that the less populous countries (Austria, Belgium, Hungary, the Netherlands, Portugal, Scandinavia, Switzerland) screen for a larger number of conditions than those with more inhabitants. That may have to do with the smaller number of professionals involved and therefore shorter lines to policymakers and ministries. Another difference is that citizens feel they are mainly a resident of their own country and not of Europe. In general, most people do not know what is happening in neighbouring countries and are also not really interested. The leverage of public opinion to put pressure on policymakers is virtually absent.

Also politically speaking, there is a difference with the US. Healthcare is one of the topics that is kept outside all treaties of the EC/EU, and is considered a national concern and responsibility. In that context, it was noticed that a resolution was adopted by the European Commission in 2008 that an exception should be made for 'rare disease'. The idea was that due to the relatively small number of patients suffering from rare diseases it would be more efficient to implement policies at a European level in the detection, diagnosis and treatment. In the ideal case, one country would focus on knowledge of one disease and another country on another disease, *etc.* It is unclear how that vision was to be implemented in practice for the care of individual patients. A result of the above decision was to make a fund available to prepare an inventory of the state of affairs concerning neonatal screening in European countries. This survey took place in 2010 and 2011 and the final report, together with a series of recommendations, was presented to the EU at the end of 2011. (Loeber *et al.*, 2013, Burgard *et al.*, 2013 Cornel *et al.*, 2014). An example of the above-mentioned large differences among countries is shown in Figure 4.2.

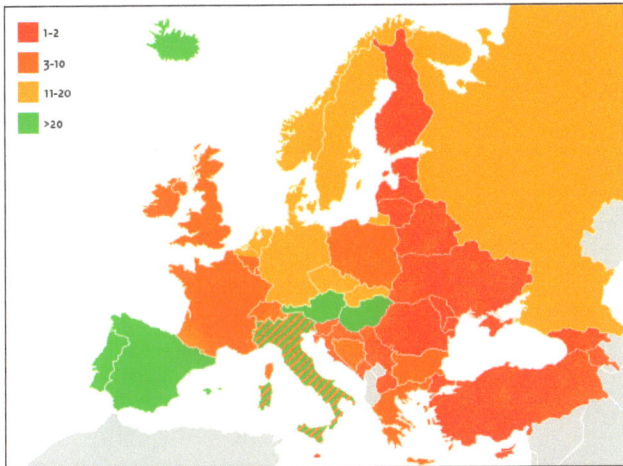

Figure 4.2. Number of diseases that are screened in a country (2011 data).

In mid-2013 it became clear (unfortunately) that the national politicians still believe that this issue should not be discussed at the European level, and that the EU currently wants to take no further concrete steps to achieve a reduction of these differences.

Situation Elsewhere

In other parts of the world, the picture is equally diverse. In Latin America, several countries (Argentina, Brazil, Uruguay) have a reasonably functioning programme, but there are also countries still at the beginning of the programme (Paraguay, Nicaragua). Asia is doing well in the United Arab Emirates, Thailand, Malaysia, the Philippines and Singapore. China pulls out all the stops to catch up; currently about 70% of the children are screened there, compared with approximately 10% only a few years ago. In India, however, with some 25 million births per year, one cannot agree on a common approach with the result that little or nothing happens. Other Asian countries are somewhere in between.

Australia and New Zealand have everything in order. Finally, in Africa, there is still much to do. Apart from Egypt and South Africa, there are only a handful of countries with some interest in neonatal screening; not surprising in light of the economic and political situation in many countries there, other health care problems require more attention.

International Associations

At an international level, several professional associations are active in order to see how they can help each other to develop programmes and harmonise a reduction to the above differences, such as the International Society for Neonatal Screening (ISNS), the Society for the Study of Inborn Errors of Metabolism (SSIEM) and the European Society for Paediatric Endocrinology (ESPE).

Chapter 5: Summary and Conclusions

Looking back over the past 40 years, a number of conclusions can be drawn. Perhaps the most important is that a screening programme can be compared to a car factory. It starts with someone with an idea, a vision, which he then shares with a few others. This is followed by sketches of the prototype, based on other existing cars, aiming to copy the strengths and deleting the weak points. After the designing phase, production follows, initially on a small scale. The number of people involved is limited; the lines of communication are short; decisions are made quickly; all stakeholders are well informed. If the first products leaving the factory are of an acceptable quality, the production is scaled up. The number of people involved increases, more people want to have a voice in decision-making, there is a hierarchy, and communication becomes more complicated. There is a need for protocols that provide a basis for resolving errors and making corrections. The production process becomes less flexible, but the product quality is stable. The original designer can then focus his attention on developing a new car.

Neonatal screening also started with a few enthusiasts (the 'designers') who became aware of the developments in the US and who thought that they might be of use in the Netherlands. They checked whom and what organisations they needed to realise their ideas and went to work in a pilot region. When the results turned out to be favourable the pilot region was extended to the whole country. It concerned only one condition, there was a relatively simple screening method and a relatively simple therapy.

Of course there were also problems encountered in practice and for which solutions had to be found. For example, thought had been given to the development of information for general practitioners and paediatricians, but not about the distribution and the associated costs; the heel prick sets would be paid by the Insurance Council, but the alcohol swabs and the Band-Aids had to be funded by privately, by the Foundation National Centre Cross. This all sounds a bit amateurish in 2014.

Incidentally, not all medical professionals were immediately convinced of the usefulness of neonatal screening of each listed condition because they felt that they could be discovered easily on the basis of clinical symptoms, thus ignoring the fact that then sometimes irreparable damage to the health of the child would have been inflicted.

Unlike the situation in a car factory, the management of the screening programme as it was organised was too weak, *i.e.* the aforementioned group of enthusiasts, united in the National Steering Committees, had the misfortune of having no mandate or decision-making powers. It was a real achievement that the LBCs functioned reasonably well from 1974 to 2003, *i.e.* 30 years!

After an interim period of three years under the wings of the Health Care Insurance Council, the screening programme matured thanks to the establishment of the Centre for Population Research (CvB) at the RIVM in 2006, as a result of a decision of the national government to take responsibility for the direction of this public health programme. The CvB came just in time to take on a very complicated big job, *i.e.* the expansion of the programme from three to 17 conditions with a large need for substantive training and some entirely new analytical techniques. The positive and negative experiences gained could be used later to instantly secure the addition of CF in 2011. For CF, the whole process was already mapped in detail; measures covering weaknesses devised, cooperation was sought from those professionals who previously had not been involved in the screening and, last but not least, solutions for financial aspects were found.

Of course it can be argued that such an approach disrupts the flexibility of the programme and that it hinders the rapid introduction of subsequent conditions, much to the chagrin of proponents of such conditions. However, the Dutch programme with this thorough approach—a strong central control with a programme committee in which all relevant professional groups and agencies are represented, and great attention to the quality of the process and the outcome—may be regarded as one of the best in the world.

Finally

A prevention programme such as neonatal screening is confection: the costs are kept low by standardising the (sub-)processes as much as possible and not changing them unnecessarily. Unfortunately, there are examples from abroad where essential processes in screening programmes were changed purely based on 'cost reduction' argumentation, without taking the risk of failure and the destruction of knowledge and experience into account. In a more market-oriented approach which is currently fashionable, special attention must be given to preserve the continuity and quality of such programmes. Therefore, at a European level, consideration should be given to keep large-scale prevention programmes outside of any free market laws promoting open competition. Let's not take any risks with the health of new borns!

Annex 1: Notes on a Number of Organisations Involved in Heel Prick Screening

Ministry and State Supervision (Ministerie en Staatstoezicht)

The Department of Health has been part of four ministries since the Second World War under different names:

1951–1971: Ministry of Social Affairs and Health (SZV)

1971–1982: Ministry of Health and Environmental Protection (VoMil)

1982–1994: Ministry of Welfare, Health and Culture (WVC)

1994–present: Ministry of Health, Welfare and Sport (VWS)

Since the Second World War, the State Supervision of Health has had various forms of Inspectorates. For the purpose of this publication, the following are important: 1951–1995: Medical Inspectorate (GHI); The Inspectorate had the following tasks:
a) Enforce laws and legal regulations in the field of public health and health care;
b) Give advice, solicited and unsolicited, from the minister in the aforementioned area;
c) Research into the state of public health and drafting of reports on this topic to the minister (Source: http://www.historici.nl, 17-06-2013).

1995–present: Health Care Inspectorate (IGZ). The Healthcare Inspectorate (IGZ) monitors public health, both in the way health care is organised and on the quality of care delivered. The Inspectorate advises the government and health care institutions. (See http://www.rijksoverheid.nl/ministeries/vws/diensten-en-instellingen).

National Institute for Public Health and the Environment (Rijksinstituut voor Volksgezondheid en Milieu)

The National Institute of Health (RIV) is part of the Ministry of Public Health. It emerged from the Central Laboratory of the Public Health Inspectorate. In 1984, RIV merged with the National Institute for Drinking Water Supply and Waste Disposal Institute to form the National Institute for Public Health and the Environment (RIVM).

The RIVM is a knowledge and research institute in the Netherlands, focusing on the promotion of public health and a healthy and safe environment. The core tasks of RIVM, performed in a national and international context, serve as policy support for the government.

The RIVM is partly responsible for providing independent and reliable information to professionals and citizens in the areas of health, medicine, environment, nutrition and safety. The aim is to exploit scientific knowledge and expertise and make it readily accessible. (See www.rivm.nl).

Cross Associations (Kruisverenigingen), Vaccination Registries (Entadministraties).

A cross association is focused on caring for the sick and wounded, and disease prevention. In the Netherlands there were the White Yellow Cross, the Green Cross and the Green-Orange Cross. They merged in 1978 into the National Cross Association. In addition, there were Provincial Cross Associations.

In the 1980s, the vaccination registries were financial departments of the Provincial Cross Association (except in Rotterdam and Amsterdam where they were part of the municipal health department).

Each Provincial Cross Association also employed what was called an MD Provincial Youth Health. This doctor was also a consultant for the Vaccination Registry. In the early 1990s the Provincial Cross Associations were dissolved. They were more or less succeeded by the Regional Home Care organisations with the National Association for Home Care as an umbrella organisation. The development of the Vaccination Registry has been described in Chapter 2.

NIPG, TNO-PG

Dutch Institute of Preventive Medicine (NIPG) in Leiden was founded in 1929 by Prof. Dr. E. Gorter. (See R. Rigter, The integration of preventive medicine into healthcare in the Netherlands (1890–1940) Gewina 19 (1996) 313–327).

In 1979 the name changed to the Dutch Institute for Preventive Health Care. Shortly thereafter, it became part of TNO. After reorganisations within TNO, the name was changed to TNO-PG. Currently it is called TNO Child Health. See further information at: www.tno.nl.

Insurance Council (Ziekenfondsraad), Health Care Insurance Board (College voor Zorgverzekeringen)

The Insurance Council was established in 1949 as supervisor of the insurance funds. Until 1999, the Insurance Council has acted as an advisory body and contributed to the creation and development of the current statutory health insurance organisations. The Insurance Council was composed of five groups: health insurance organisations, employers, employees, healthcare professionals and ministerial officials. The Insurance Council gave the Minister advice on new care facilities such as the feasibility of new screening programs.

In 1996, the Minister decided that the model of participation had to be replaced by a model of exclusively independent experts. To emphasize that, the name was changed to the Health Care Insurance Board.

Health Council (Gezondheidsraad)

The Health Council has been, since 1902, an independent scientific advisory body. Its task is to advise the government and Parliament in the field of public health issues and health (services) research. This field also traditionally includes such topics as nutrition, environmental protection and occupational hygiene and, for some years, assessing license applications for medical screening. One of the current six focus areas is Prevention, i.e. advising on screening and vaccination. Most of the advice given by the Health Council is written at the request of one of the ministers. With some regularity, the Health Council publishes unsolicited opinions that have a signalling function. In some cases, this advice leads to a minister requesting further advice further on the topic. (See www.gezondheidsraad.nl).

Annex 2: Persons Who Have Contributed

Supervisory Committee Members

Prof. Dr. M.C. Cornel, MD, chair Programmacommissie Neonatale Hielprikscreening, VUmc, Amsterdam

Dr. W.J. Dondorp, ethicist, Universiteit Maastricht

Prof. Dr. E.S. Houwaart, medical historian, Universiteit Maastricht

Mr. A. Lock, MD, medical advisor RIVM-CvB

Mrs. H. Meutgeert, director Vereniging Volwassenen, Kinderen en Stofwisselingsziekten

Dr. G.C.M.L. Page-Christiaens, gynaecologist, chair Gezondheidsraadcommissie Neonatale Screening 2003–2005, UMC Utrecht

Prof. D.B. Paul, ethicist, University of Massachusetts Boston, USA

Dr. M. Prins, policymaker Ministry VWS

Prof. Dr. F.J. van Spronsen, paediatrician, chair Adviescommissie Metabole Ziekten

Dr. P.H. Verkerk, MD, epidemiologist, TNO

Interviews

Dr. H. Cohen, MD, former Director-General RIVM

Dr. E.H.B.M. Dekkers, programme coordinator neonatale hielprikscreening RIVM-CvB

Dr. G. Derksen-Lubsen, paediatrician, chair LBC-CH 1992–2003

Dr. P.C. Groeneveld, policy maker Ministerie VWS

Prof. Dr. G.A. de Jonge, paediatrician, voorzitter LBC-CH 1975–1992

Mr. A. Lock, arts, medical advisor RIVM-CvB

Mrs. H. Meutgeert, director Vereniging Volwassenen, Kinderen en Stofwisselingsziekten

Mrs. M. Oey-Sprauwen, MD, medical advisor RIVM-DVP

Dr. M. Prins, policy maker Ministerie VWS

Dr. J. Rechsteiner, MD, microbiologist, head RIVM screenings laboratory 1979–1984

Dr. W. Schopman, clinical chemist, head reference laboratory CH, 1979–1990

Prof. Dr. F.J. van Sprang, paediatrician, chair LBC-PKU 1974–1985

Prof. Dr. F.J. van Spronsen, paediatrician, chair Adviescommissie Metabole Ziekten

Dr. H.P. Verbrugge, MD, former Inspector Health Care

Dr. P.H. Verkerk, MD, epidemiologist, TNO

Prof. Dr. H.K.A. Visser, paediatrician -endocrinologist

Dr. C.E. Voogd, biologist, head reference laboratory PKU 1968–1992

Others

Mr. L.H. Elvers, head RIVM screening laboratory 1996–2012
Dr. B. Hoebee, biochemist, head RIVM CvB
Dr. P.C.J.I. Schielen, medical biologist, head RIVM reference laboratory 2012–today
Mr. P.A.A.M. de Hoogh, advisor RIVM-DVP
Mrs. Y.H.H.M. Wijnands, MD, medical advisor RIVM-DVP

Annex 3: Referenced Documents, Scientific Literature and Internet Sources

Anders GJP, van Duyne WMJ, Fleury P, Hartgerink MJ, Hoejenbos E, Tegelaers WHM, Voogd CE, Zijlstra R (1973) The prevalence of phenylketonuria patients in Dutch institutes for the mentally retarded in 1968. Bulletin van de Coördinatiecommissie Biochemisch Onderzoek van de sectie psychiatrische instituten van de Nationale Ziekenhuisraad 6: 35–39.

van den Berg M (2007) Je moet niet alles willen weten. Leidsch Dagblad 12-01-2007.

Bergink AH (1976) PKU-screening. Maandblad voor Verzorging, Opvoeding, Onderwijs, 11: 248-250.

Bongers-Schokking JG, van den Brande JL, Derksen-Lubsen G, Drayer NM, Gons MH, Tegelaers WHH, de Vijlder JJM, eds. (1980) Screening op congenitale hypothyreoïdie. Werkmap voor kinderartsen, 1^e uitgave (1986 2^e uitgave) Leiden:NIPG-TNO.

Bovenberg JA (2006) Property Rights in Blood, Genes and Data; naturally yours? PhD thesis Leiden University.

van den Burg S, Verweij M (2012) Maintaining Trust in Newborn Screening. Hastings Center Report 42: 41–47.

Burgard P, Rupp K, Lindner M, Haege G, Rigter T, Weinreich SS, Loeber JG, Taruscio D, Vittozzi L, Cornel MC, Hoffmann GF (2012) Newborn screening programmes in Europe; arguments and efforts regarding harmonization. Part 2 – From screening laboratory results to treatment, follow-up and quality assurance. J Inher Metab Dis 35: 613–625.

Centerwall WR (1957). Phenylketonuria. J.Am.Med.Ass. 165: 392, 2219.

Cornel MC, Rigter T, Weinreich SS, Burgard P, Hoffmann GF, Lindner M, Loeber JG, Rupp K, Taruscio D, Vittozzi L (2014) A framework to start the debate on neonatal screening policies in the EU: an Expert Opinion Document. Eur.J.Hum.Genet. 22: 12-17.

Derks TGJ (2007) MCAD Deficiency, Clinical and laboratory studies. PhD thesis Groningen University.

Derksen-Lubsen G (1981) Screening for Congenital Hypothyroidism in The Netherlands. PhD thesis Erasmus University Rotterdam.

Derksen-Lubsen G, de Jonge GA (1978) Aangeboren Schildklierstoornis: Onderzoek van pasgeborenen. TNO, Leiden.

Detmar S, Dijkstra N, Nijsingh N, Rijnders M, Verweij M, Hosli E. (2008) Parental opinions about the expansion of the neonatal screening programme. Commun. Genetics 11: 11–17.

Directeur-Generaal Volksgezondheid (1972) Brief aan Geneeskundig Hoofdinspecteur betreffende Advies inzake rapport Studiegroep Phenylketonurie, nr 85234 10-11-1972. Nationaal Archief Den Haag, inventarisnummer 2.15.65/320.

Draaiboek Phenylketonurie-PKU (1973) Werkgroep PKU. Geneeskundige Hoofdinspectie van de Volksgezondheid, Leidschendam.

Dussault JH, Laberge C (1973) Thyroxine (T4) determination by radioimmunological method in dried blood eluate: new diagnostic method of neonatal hypothyroidism? Union Med Can. 102: 2062–2064.

Elvers LH, Diependaal GAM, Blonk J, Loeber JG (1995) Phenylketonuria screening using the Quantase phenylalaninekit in combination with a microfilter system and the dye Tartrazine. Screening 3: 209–223.

Elvers LH, Loeber JG, Boelen A, Kemper-Proper EA, Rondeel JMM, Triepels RH (2008–2012) Neonatale hielprikscreening. Jaaroverzichten screeningslaboratoria 2008–2012. RIVM rapporten.

Erfocentrum (2014) Aandoeningen en erfelijkheid http://www.erfocentrum.nl/ voorlichtingsmateriaal 13-01-2014.

Fisher DA (2005) Next generation newborn screening for congenital hypothyroidism? J Clin Endocrinol Metab 90: 3797–3799.

Fleury P (1959) Oligophrenia Phenylpyruvica. PhD thesis Utrecht University.

Følling A (1934) Über Ausscheidung von Phenylbrenztraubensäure in den Harn als Stoffwechselanomalie in Verbindung mit Imbezillität. Hoppe-Seyler´s Zeitschrift für physiologische Chemie 227: 169–181.

Garrod AE (1909) Inborn Errors of Metabolism, reprinted in Garrod's Inborn Errors of Metabolism, with a supplement by H. Harris (London: Oxford University Press, 1963).

Geneeskundige Hoofdinspectie (1974) GHI-Bulletin Phenylketonurie.

Geneeskundige Hoofdinspectie (1980) GHI-Bulletin Congenitale Hypothyreoïdie.

Gezondheidsraad (1979) Screening op aangeboren stofwisselingsziekten. Gezondheidsraad, publicatie nr. 1979/7.

Gezondheidsraad (1989) Erfelijkheid: wetenschap en maatschappij. Gezondheidsraad, publicatie nr. 1989/31.

Gezondheidsraad (1994) Genetische screening. Gezondheidsraad, publicatie nr. 1994/22.

Gezondheidsraad (2003a) Neonatale screening met behulp van massaspectrometrie. Verslag van een door de Gezondheidsraad belegde workshop. Gezondheidsraad, 2003.

Gezondheidsraad (2003b) Signalering Ethiek en Gezondheid 2003. Gezondheidsraad publicatie nr. 2003/08.

Gezondheidsraad (2005) Neonatale screening. Gezondheidsraad, publicatie nr. 2005/11.

Gezondheidsraad (2010) Neonatale screening op cystic fibrosis. Gezondheidsraad, publicatie nr. 2010/01.

Gezondheidsraad (2010b) Het 'duizend dollar genoom': een ethische verkenning. Gezondheidsraad, publicatie nr. 2010/15.

Guthrie R, Susi A (1963) A simple phenylalanine method for detecting phenylketonuria in large populations of newborn infants. Pediatrics 32: 338–343.

Hermans H (1974) PKU-onderzoek negen maanden vertraagd. Maandblad voor de Zwakzinnigenzorg KLIK 7: 2 en 32.

Holtzman NA, Mellits ED, Kallman CH (1974) Neonatal screening for phenylketonuria. II. Age dependence of initial phenylalanine in infants with PKU. Pediatrics. 53: 353–357.

Huisman J, Slijper FME, Hendrikx MMT, Kalverboer AF, van der Schot L (1985) Intelligentie van vroeg-behandelde patiënten met phenylketonurie, 10 jaar psychologische follow-up in Nederland. Ned Tijdschr Geneesk. 129: 2120–2123.

Kalverboer AF, Bleeker JK (1988) De mentale en psychomotorische ontwikkeling van bij vroege screening ontdekte patiëntjes met congenitale hypothyreoïdie. Ned Tijdschr Geneeskd. 132: 539–543.

van der Kamp HJ (2001) Congenital drenal hyperplasia: treatment and neonatal screening. PhD thesis Leiden University.

ten Kate LP, Loeber JG, de Knijf P, Bovenberg JA (2005) Trends in onze genen. Med.Contact 60: 1767–1769.

Kemper-Proper EA, Elvers LH, Loeber JG (2009) De nieuwe hielprikscreening vanuit de screeningslaboratoria: ervaringen en lessen na één jaar. Ned.Tijdschr.Klin.Chem. Labgeneesk. 34: 189–196.

Koch R, Gross Friedman E, Wenz E, Jew K, Crowley C, Donnell G (1986) Maternal Phenylketonuria. J.Inher.Metab.Dis. 9, Suppl.2: 159–168.

de Koning HJ, Juttmann RE, Panman J, Verzijl JG, Meulmeester JF, van Oortmarssen GJ *et al*. (1992) Kosten-effectiviteitsanalyse in dejeugdgezondheidszorg voor 0–4-jarigen: methode en mogelijkheden. Instituut Maatschappelijke Gezondheidszorg, Erasmus Universiteit Rotterdam,1992.

Landelijke Begeleidingscommissie Phenylketonurie (1978) De vroege opsporing van fenylketonurie in Nederland in de periode 1 september 1974-31 december 1976. Ned. Tijdschr. Geneesk. 41: 1558–1562.

Landelijke Begeleidingscommissie Phenylketonurie (1981) De vroege opsporing van fenylketonurie in Nederland 1977–1979. Ned. Tijdschr. Geneesk. 125: 2135–2140.

Lanting CI, van Tijn DA, Loeber JG, Vulsma T, de Vijlder JJM, Verkerk PH (2005) Clinical Effectiveness and Cost-Effectiveness of the Use of the Thyroxine/Thyroxine-Binding Globulin Ratio to Detect Congenital Hypothyroidism of Thyroidal and Central Origin in a Neonatal Screening Programme. Pediatrics 116: 168–173.

Loeber JG (2000) De opslag van hielprikkaarten: feiten en fabels. Tijdschr.Verlosk. 25: 868–891.

Loeber JG, Elvers LH, Endert E., van Landeghem AAJ, Rondeel JMM, Verheul FEAM (1990–2007) Jaarrapporten Landelijke screening op phenylketonurie, congenitale hypothyreoidie en adrenogenitaal syndroom. RIVM rapporten.

Loeber JG, Burgard P, Cornel MC, Rigter T, Weinreich SS, Rupp K, Hoffmann GF, Vittozzi L (2012) Newborn screening programmes in Europe; arguments and efforts regarding harmonization. Part 1 – From blood spot to screening result. J Inher Metab Dis 35: 603–611.

Loeber JG (1986) Verkennend onderzoek naar de mogelijkheden tot (verdere) automatisering van de uitslagverwerking van de PKU/CHT screening. RIVM rapport nr. 368104008.

Loeber JG (1987) Voorbereiding van de (verdere) automatisering van de uitslagverwerking van de PKU/CHT screening. RIVM rapport nr. 368104009.

Manten A (1964) Nota aan Directie RIV betreffende Opsporing van fenylketonurie bij zeer jonge zuigelingen, nr U 537/64 Chemo Ma/gvo. Persoonlijk archief drs CE Voogd.

Manten A, Holtz AH (1964) Brief aan JJL ten Brink, Psychiatrische Inrichting Voorburg te Vught, nr U 122/64 Chemo Ma/mvd inzake start PKU-preventie. Persoonlijk archief drs CE Voogd.

Manten A, Voogd CE (1968) Opsporing van fenylketonurie in inrichtingen. RIV rapport 91/68.

Meijer WJ (1985) Tien jaar landelijk screeningsonderzoek naar het vóórkomen van fenylketonurie in Nederland; derde verslag van de Landelijke Begeleidingscommissie Phenylketonurie. Ned.Tijdschr. Geneesk. 129: 74–76.

Nationaal Orgaan Zwakzinnigenzorg (1974) Laat zelf al een PKU-onderzoek doen en stuur de rekening naar uw ziekenfonds. Maandblad voor de Zwakzinnigenzorg KLIK 7: 25–26.

National Aacademy of Sciences (1975) Genetic Screening. Report of the Committee for the study of inborn errors of metabolism, Washington DC.

Nelck GF (1965) Capita Selecta – Phenylketonurie. Ned.Tijdschr.Geneesk. 109: 1115–1121.

Niermeijer MF, de Koning TJ, Meutgeert HK (2007) Neonatale Screening te snel uitgebreid. Medisch Contact 10: 416–418.

Otten BJ (1987) Salivary 17-OH progesterone and androstenedione in congential adrenal hyperplasia. PhD thesis Nijmegen University.

van der Pal S, Otten W, Detmar S (2010) Evaluatie van de voorlichting aan ouders over de hielprik. Tijdschr. Soc. Geneesk. 88: 449–453.

Paul DB, Brosco JP (2013) The PKU Paradox, a short history of a genetic disease. John Hopkins University Press, Baltimore, USA.

Peters M, Appel IM, Cnossen MH, Breuning-Boers JM, Heijboer H (2009) Sikkelcelziekte in de hielprikscreening. I. Ned.Tijdschr.Geneeskd. 153: B359.

Plass AMC, van El CG, Pieters T, Cornel MC. (2010) Neonatal screening for treatable and untreatable disorders: Prospective parents' opinion in the Netherlands. Pediatrics 125: 99–106.

van der Putten A, Wiegers T (2005) Evaluatie van het functioneren van het hielprikprogramma: de neonatale screening op phenylketonurie, congenitale hypothyreoïdie en het adrenogenitaal syndroom. NIVEL Utrecht.

Rechsteiner J (1979) Mechanisering en automatisering van serologische bepalingen, Spaander Symposium 11-12-1979, pag 25–29, RIVM Bilthoven.

Reerink A (2007) Ouders ziek kind willen hielprik, geen roze wolk. NRC 04-01-2007.

RIVM (2014a) Criteria van Wilson&Jungner http://www.rivm.nl/Onderwerpen/B/ Bevolkingsonderzoeken_en_screeningen/Achtergrondinformatie/Screening_de_theorie/Criter ia_voor_verantwoorde_screening 29-01-2014.

RIVM (2014b) De ziektes die de hielprik opspoort, http://www.rivm.nl/Onderwerpen/H/ Hielprik/De_ziektes_die_de_hielprik_opspoort , 13-01-2014.

RIVM (2014c) Draaiboek Neonatale Hielprikscreening http://www.rivm.nl/Documenten_en_ publicaties/Professioneel_Praktisch/Draaiboeken/Preventie_Ziekte_Zorg/Hielprik/Draaiboek _Neonatale_Hielprikscreening_v_9_1, 13-01-2014.

Schipper HS (2008) Genetic Screening and Patient Autonomy. The theory and practice of informed decision making. PhD thesis Groningen University.

Schopman W (1981–1990) Kwartaalrapporten over de analytische vergelijking van de CHT-laboratoria. Referentielaboratorium CHT, Bergwegziekenhuis, Rotterdam, in opdracht van RIVM.

van Sprang FJ (1961) Fenylketonurie. PhD thesis Utrecht University.

Staatssecretaris Volksgezondheid&Milieuhygiëne (1974) Besluit uitvoering onderzoek aangeboren stofwisselingsziekten Bijzondere ziektekostenverzekering nr 84614 plus Brief aan DG RIV 26-06-1974. Nationaal Archief Den Haag, inventarisnummer 2.15.65/641.

Studiegroep Phenylketonurie (1970) Rapport inventarisatie kennis over phenylketonurie en mogelijkheden tot opsporing. Nationaal Archief Den Haag, inventarisnummer 2.27.5310/4657.

Swaak AJ (1976) De Phenylketonuriescreening en de voeding van de zuigeling. Medisch Contact 31: 13–14.

Swaak AJ (1978) Oneigenlijk gebruik van bloedmonsters? Medisch Contact 33: 1027–1028.

Tijmstra TJ (1984) Betekenis van een vals-positieve uitslag bij neonatale screeningsprogramma's. Tijdschr Soc Gezondheidsz 62: 447–449.

Tijmstra TJ, Tjeerdema H, Pennings JM, Smit GPA (2008) Ouders stellen nauwelijks grenzen aan de hielprik. Tijdschr Kindergeneesk 76: 23–26.

Vansenne F, de Borgie CAJM, Bouva MJ, Legdeur MA, van Zwieten R, Petrij F, Peters M (2009) Sikkelcelziekte in de hielprikscreening. II. Ned.Tijdschr.Geneeskd. 153: B366.

Veraart JBM (1965) Brief aan Directie RIV met herhaalde vraag om aandacht voor PKU screening, d.d. 18-06-1965. Nationaal Archief Den Haag, inventarisnummer 2.27.5310/4973.

Verbrugge HP (1983) Fenylketonurie; screening van pasgeborenen een juist besluit? Med Contact 31: 958–960.

Verkerk PH en diverse co-auteurs (1991–2012) Evaluate van de hielprikscreening bij kinderen geboren in kalenderjaren 1990–2011, TNO Leiden.

Verkerk PH, Derksen-Lubsen G, Vulsma T, Loeber JG, de Vijlder JJM, Verbrugge HP (1993) Evaluatie van een decennium neonatale screening op congenitale hypothyreoidie in Nederland. Ned Tijdschr Geneeskd 137: 2199–2205.

Verkerk PH (1995) Twintig jaar landelijke screening op fenyl-ketonurie in Nederland. Ned Tijdschr Geneeskd 139: 2302–2305.

Vernooij-van Langen AMM (2013) Newborn Screening for cystic fibrosis in the Netherlands; the CHOPIN study. PhD thesis Maastricht University.

Visser G. van Spronsen FJ, de Sain-van der Velden MG, Blom HJ, Wijburg FA (2009) Uitgebreide neonatale hielprikscreening op stofwisselingsziekten in Nederland. Ned.Tijdschr.Geneeskd. 153: B360.

Voogd CE (1973) Iets over fenylketonurie. Tijdschr. Praktische Verloskunde 77: 173–175, plus naschrift in Tijdschr. Praktische Verloskunde 78: 107.

Voogd CE (1973) Phenylketonurie, waar gaat het om? Maatschappelijke Gezondheidszorg 12: 794–797.

Voogd CE (1974) Opsporing van erfelijke ziekten door middel van bevolkingsonderzoek. Maandschr. Kindergeneesk. 42: 9–17.

Voogd CE (1974) Opsporing van fenylketonurie in Nederland. Tijdschr. Med.Analisten 29: 253–264.

VSOP (Vereniging Samenwerkende Ouder- en Patiëntenorganisaties) (1999). Neonatale screening op aandoeningen waarvoor geen medische behandeling is. In: Poortman Y, red. Genetisch onderzoek. Mensen, meningen en medeverantwoordelijkheid. Baarn, Fontein; p. 106–11.

de Vries HG, Niezen-Koning K, Kliphuis JW, Smit GP, Scheffer H, ten Kate LP (1996) Prevalence of carriers of the most common medium-chain acyl-CoA dehydrogenase (MCAD) deficiency mutation (G985A) in The Netherlands. Hum Genet. 98: 1–2.

Vulsma T (1991) Etiology and pathogenesis of congenital hypothyroidism, PhD thesis Amsterdam University.

Waelkens JJJ (1989) Osteomyelitis van de calcaneus bij pasgeborenen; wie is bang voor een prikje? Ned Tijdschr Geneesk. 133: 1641–1644.

Watson M, Mann MY, Lloyd-Puryear MA, Rinaldo P, Howell RR (2006) Newborn screening: toward a uniform screening panel and system – executive summary. Pediatrics 117: S296–S307.

Weinreich SS, Rigter T, van El CG, Dondorp WJ, Kostense PJ, van der Ploeg AT, Reuser AJ, Cornel MC, Hagemans ML (2012) Public support for neonatal screening for Pompe disease, a broad-phenotype condition. Orphanet J Rare Dis. 7:15.

de Wert, GMWR (2005) Cascade screening: whose information is it anyway? Eur. J. Human Genetics 13: 397–398.

Wilson JM, Jungner YG (1968) Principles and practice of mass screening for disease. Bull WHO 65: 281–393.

Yalow RS, Berson SA (1960) Immunoassay of endogenous plasma insulin in man. J Clin Invest. 39: 1157–1175.

Annex 4: References of Illustrations

1.1.	Courtesy Museum of disABILITY History, Buffalo (NY), USA
1.2.	Drs C.E.Voogd, personal archive
1.3.	National Archive Den Haag, inventarisnummer 2.15.65/641
1.4.	Dr H.P.Verbrugge, personal archive
1.5.	Archive Landelijke Begeleidingscommissie CH
1.6.	Based on data from Verkerk *et al.* (1991–2012)
1.7.	Archive Landelijke Begeleidingscommissie CH
1.8.	Based on data from Verkerk *et al.* (1991–2012)
1.9.	Publication Centrum voor Bevolkingsonderzoek RIVM
2.1.	Courtesy Centrum voor Bevolkingsonderzoek RIVM
2.2.	Courtesy Dienst Vaccinaties en Preventieprogramma's RIVM
2.3.	Archive Landelijke Begeleidingscommissie CH
2.4.	Archive Landelijke Begeleidingscommissie CH
2.5.	Publication Centrum voor Bevolkingsonderzoek RIVM
2.6.	Dr J.G. Loeber, personal archive
2.7.	Journal Trouw 19 mei 2000, www.trouw.nl
2.8.	Various journals period 13–23 May 2000
2.9.	Various journals November 2000
2.10.	Dr J.G. Loeber, personal archive
3.1.	Courtesy Centrum voor Bevolkingsonderzoek RIVM
3.2.	Dr J.G. Loeber, personal archive
3.3.	Courtesy Centrum voor Bevolkingsonderzoek RIVM
3.4.	Photocollection RIVM
3.5.	Photocollection RIVM
3.6.	Photocollection RIVM
3.7.	Photocollection RIVM
4.1.	Based on data from Loeber *et al.* (2012)
4.2.	Based on data from Loeber *et al.* (2012)

MDPI AG
Klybeckstrasse 64
4057 Basel, Switzerland
Tel. +41 61 683 77 34
Fax +41 61 302 89 18
http://www.mdpi.com

MDPI Books
E-mail: books@mdpi.com
http://books.mdpi.com